Praise for *The Unexpected*

"They don't sugarcoat reality, and they make great use of statistics. . . . Oster and Fox want to arm moms with information about what they should ask their providers and what treatments might lower their risks in subsequent pregnancies. . . . The message from these compassionate authors, parents themselves, is that what happened needs to be processed, not ignored, and joy is still possible." —Karen Springen, *Booklist*

"Encouraging and empathetic . . . On every page, the authors offer extensive research and support. . . . A comprehensive, empowering resource." —*Kirkus Reviews*

"Cogent . . . Informative but not dry. It's a valuable resource for parents who have experienced pregnancy complications." —*Publishers Weekly*

T0370116

PENGUIN BOOKS

THE UNEXPECTED

Emily Oster is a professor of economics at Brown University and the author of *The Family Firm: A Data-Driven Guide to Better Decision Making in the Early School Years*; *Cribsheet: A Data-Driven Guide to Better, More Relaxed Parenting, from Birth to Preschool*; and *Expecting Better: Why the Conventional Pregnancy Wisdom Is Wrong—and What You Really Need to Know*. She writes the newsletter *ParentData*, and her work has been featured in *The New York Times*, *The Wall Street Journal*, *The Washington Post*, *The Atlantic*, and Bloomberg.com. She has two children.

Dr. Nathan Fox is a professor of obstetrics and gynecology and maternal-fetal medicine at the Icahn School of Medicine at Mount Sinai in New York City. He has a busy clinical practice of high-risk obstetrics, regularly publishes his peer-reviewed clinical research, and is invited to lecture nationally and internationally on pregnancy-related topics. He is also the host of the *Healthful Woman* podcast. He has four children.

Also by Emily Oster

Expecting Better

Cribsheet

The Family Firm

The
Unexpected

Navigating Pregnancy
During and After Complications

EMILY OSTER

AND NATHAN FOX, MD

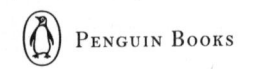 PENGUIN BOOKS

PENGUIN BOOKS
An imprint of Penguin Random House LLC
1745 Broadway, New York, NY 10019
penguinrandomhouse.com

Set in Dante MT Std
Designed by Cassandra Garruzzo Mueller

ISBN 9780593831229 (paperback)

THE LIBRARY OF CONGRESS HAS CATALOGED THE HARDCOVER EDITION AS FOLLOWS:
Names: Oster, Emily, author. | Fox, Nathan (Physician), author.
Title: The unexpected : navigating pregnancy during and
after complications / Emily Oster and Nathan Fox, MD.
Description: New York : Penguin Press, 2024. |
Includes bibliographical references and index.
Identifiers: LCCN 2023038447 (print) | LCCN 2023038448 (ebook) |
ISBN 9780593652770 (hardcover) | ISBN 9780593652787 (ebook)
Subjects: LCSH: Subsequent pregnancy. | Pregnancy—Health aspects. |
Pregnant women—Health and hygiene. | Prenatal care.
Classification: LCC RG525 .O87 2024 (print) | LCC RG525 (ebook) |
DDC 618.2—dc23/eng/20231214
LC record available at https://lccn.loc.gov/2023038447
LC ebook record available at https://lccn.loc.gov/2023038448

First published in the United States of America by Penguin Press,
an imprint of Penguin Random House LLC, 2024
Published in Penguin Books 2025

Printed in the United States of America
1st Printing

The authorized representative in the EU for product safety and compliance is
Penguin Random House Ireland, Morrison Chambers, 32 Nassau Street,
Dublin D02 YH68, Ireland, https://eu-contact.penguin.ie.

This book is dedicated to all of the people who inspired it—to those who trusted their stories with me, especially the hard ones.

—Emily Oster

To Michal, for always being my biggest fan. I love you.

—Nathan Fox

Contents

PART 1

Preparation

Complications

Post-Birth Complications

Introduction

I remember vividly the moment I decided to write a book about pregnancy. I was 10 weeks pregnant with my first child. I was at my first real prenatal visit, and the one topic I knew we needed to discuss was prenatal testing. I had some idea of the two options available at the time—an ultrasound-based screening procedure or a more invasive, but more accurate, test—and I was ready to dive into which might be the best for my pregnancy.

Instead of the discussion I expected, I was told simply that the ultrasound procedure was the appropriate option, given my age. When I tried to push back—surely more factors were relevant than *just* age— I was told begrudgingly that if necessary I could investigate the second option. But, they emphasized, it was really nonstandard and I would have to make a decision within a few days. On my own.

I ended up, thirty minutes after the appointment, standing on a street corner in Chicago, on the phone with my husband, trying to work out what information we needed to figure this out. I spent the next several days furiously working through academic papers, datasets, and spreadsheets to try to figure out what we should do.

What I took from this, above all, was a feeling of being *unprepared*. I was ready, emotionally, to engage in this question. But I didn't have the necessary information or the right way to approach the conversation. The discussions I had with my doctor, on this and other topics, were challenging in large part because I didn't have enough information to enter them with the right questions.

I spent much of that first pregnancy trying to figure out how to ask the right questions and to find the data to inform the choices that I had to make. *Expecting Better*, the book that the pregnancy inspired, was my attempt to fix this problem for other people. Yes, much of that book is about lifestyle choices—important ones, like whether you can have sushi or coffee. But a big portion is about previewing the medical choices you'll have to make and walking through the information needed to make them, or at least to engage in productive conversations about them.

When I got to my second pregnancy, I was in a very different position. This was partly because I had written a book about pregnancy. It was also because I was very lucky. My first pregnancy was smooth. Very few new questions arose before the second. I had no significant complications previously that I felt I needed to prepare for.

This is not true for everyone. If people largely come into their first pregnancy with similar expectations, we all come into a second (or third, or fourth) pregnancy with the weight of our different experiences, good or bad. When these experiences are complicated, the landscape going forward is complicated, too.

This isn't a rare or niche problem. Complicated pregnancies affect a lot of us. If we put together all of the conditions discussed in this book—miscarriage, preterm birth, preeclampsia, hyperemesis gravidarum, and many more—we are talking about perhaps 50 percent of pregnancies. And that means that as much as half of our later pregnancies carry this extra layer of difficulty.

I wrote *Expecting Better* more than a decade ago. In that time, I have continued to work as a professor specializing in health economics and statistical methods. I have also written two other books, as well as countless issues of a newsletter, *ParentData*, about pregnancy and parenting. Through this work, through emails, DMs, research, surveys, and personal interactions, I have had the privilege to see an enormous range of pregnancy experience.

People write for help with navigating pregnancy after loss. Once, a reader wrote to share the heartbreaking news that she had lost her son at 20 weeks. She was looking for answers, which I'm sorry to say I didn't really have at the time. Then, a couple of years later, she wrote to me again, this time sharing pictures of her new baby.

People write for help with treatments—*I had preeclampsia before—should I take aspirin this time?*

They write for reassurance. *My doctor said this complication is really unlikely to happen again but . . . is that right?*

They write to share their complicated decision making around future pregnancies. *I want to give my son a sibling but I'm just not sure I can do that again.*

I feel the sadness that can come through some of these emails, but also the joy that's sometimes on the other side. I feel privileged to be with them for a portion of what can be an incredibly challenging time. I feel lucky when I can help, and frustrated when I cannot.

Ultimately, when people reached out to me with these questions about pregnancy after complications, they were almost always looking for data. They had been through an experience that was incredibly emotionally fraught, and they were trying to make the best decision possible and move forward. People craved evidence, something to help them process and contextualize what they had experienced and what it might mean for the future.

What I also heard, along with a desire for data, was a much more intense version of the same feeling I had during my first prenatal visit. Navigating or planning a pregnancy after complications can plunge you into an unfamiliar world of medical decision making. Conversations with medical providers can be hard and scary, and often people felt that they were given a choice about what to do without really having the full set of information they needed, or they weren't given any choices at all.

Data is one important input, but another key is knowing the right questions. In so many of the scenarios we'll talk about in this book, the right decision depends on the particulars of your situation. Your medical provider will be the key partner in figuring this out, which makes it all the more important that those provider conversations are as constructive as possible. That will be easier if you're coming into the office with more knowledge, with a better sense of the right set of questions.

I wrote this book to try to help people navigate these crucial moments of their lives. This goal—to empower people to make better, more confident decisions in their pregnancy and parenting—imbues everything I do in my writing. It's the reason I write every day, and the thing that I love. In that sense, this book is no different from my existing work.

What is different about this book is that I hope you do not have to read it. It is odd to write a book that you hope people will not need. I very much want people to read my other books, but this one, I wish you would be able to pass by.

However, I go back to the reality just discussed. Twenty-five percent of pregnancies end in miscarriage. Five to 10 percent of women will be diagnosed with diabetes or preeclampsia. Approximately 10 percent of births are preterm. We do not talk about this, and yet there it is. These issues affect an enormous number of pregnancies.

The lack of discussion is part of the problem. So many of the conditions experienced here are kept quiet, or secret. The secrecy of miscarriage we are perhaps aware of. But it goes beyond this. How many of us know the details of even our close friend's vaginal tearing or uterine prolapse? How frequently do you hear people discuss the experience of a child spending a month in the NICU, or the details of postpartum anxiety? Hiding these things can leave us feeling alone. That loneliness compounds an already painful situation.

It also discourages necessary research and policy discussion. There are many places in this book where we'll come to conclusions along the lines of "We don't really know what works here," even when it seems like learning what works could be within reach. But research funding often follows public discussions, and public discussions cannot happen if we are not willing to talk about these hard things.

So, this book has three goals.

First, to bring these maternal health complications into the light. As I said, I hope no one needs to read this book for themselves, but I hope everyone reads it to better understand the experiences of others.

Second, to give those of you who do need this book the data you have been asking for. For each complication, I'm going to try hard to answer two key questions: What is the risk of recurrence in a later pregnancy? And what treatments might lower that risk? This second question will usually prompt a third: How can I better prepare if it does happen again?

Third, to give people an avenue toward more productive conversations with their providers. Data will help, but to make these hard talks as useful as possible, you need a script—a way to be prepared to get the information you need, and a way to structure the conversation. You need to have some understanding of how your provider is thinking about your situation so that together you arrive at the best possible result. Having productive conversations with your provider is key to that end.

I couldn't achieve this third goal on my own. So I brought in an expert in this space: Dr. Nathan Fox, a maternal-fetal medicine specialist at Mount Sinai in New York City. Nate will wear many hats in this book—he's a key contributor to the medical details throughout. His input is integrated into many of the data sections, just as I had input from medical editors in prior books. And, once you have the data on recurrence and treatment from me, he'll end each chapter with thoughts from his side of the table based on his experience and expertise about how to move forward with your medical provider in light of these realities.

He'll give insight into how to best approach these conversations. Nate has treated thousands of patients over his career, and he's seen the many different courses these complex scenarios can take.

This book is a true collaboration (something that was hard for me, given my control tendencies—personal growth!). In nearly all cases, it was immediately clear to me why it was so important to bring the data together with a detailed medical perspective. The questions here are complicated and nuanced. They rarely have easy answers just based on the data. The challenge is about finding what is right *for you*, rather than looking for what *is right*.

With that, I will let Nate introduce himself.

I am an OB-GYN and maternal-fetal medicine (MFM) specialist practicing in New York City. I was born and raised in Chicago and then came out to New York for college, met my wife, and never left the city, at least professionally. I went to medical school at Mount Sinai in New York, stayed there for my OB-GYN residency, went twenty blocks away to NewYork-Presbyterian/Cornell for my MFM fellowship, and then returned to a private practice at Mount Sinai called Maternal Fetal Medicine Associates, where I have been ever since. My wife and I live in New Jersey now, and we have four children, one son-in-law, and two dogs.

As a doctor, I see patients every day, either in the office for prenatal care, consultations, ultrasounds, or fetal procedures, or when I'm on the labor floor delivering babies. By nature I am social, so my passion has always been spending time with patients and their families, getting to know them and trying to help them through complicated (or not complicated) pregnancies. On the side, I've always had an academic curiosity, so after my fellowship I continued to participate in medical research in areas such as twin pregnancies, preterm birth, and ultrasound.

A few years ago, I came to the realization that despite the explosion in online content, it was actually becoming harder for women to get reliable information about pregnancy and health care in general. It was difficult to navigate the sea of information and find information that was accurate but also relevant to your specific question or concern.

This led me to start my podcast, *Healthful Woman*. At the same time, in around 2017, one of my patients recommended a book on pregnancy, *Expecting Better*, written by an economist, Emily Oster. The patient told me the book read like something I could have written, and she was correct! I loved it, reached out to Emily, and we have been collaborating ever since. So it was only natural that we would write a book together, and I am very excited we are doing so.

My role in this book is complementary to Emily's. Emily is a master information gatherer, sifter, and teacher. She is able to give you tremendous insight into a wide variety of topics and how to approach them yourself and with your doctor or midwife. I hope to uncover for you how your doctor may be approaching your situation or your questions. If you are trying to plan for a pregnancy, it is best to come prepared with your own thoughts on the subject, but also with an understanding of what your doctor is thinking. This can hopefully allow you, and your doctor, to have the most productive and personalized conversation possible about what might be best for you given your specific needs, background, and health history.

In all medical decisions, there is a balance between the doctor making a decision or recommendation and your choosing the right option for yourself. I specify that it is a "balance" because how much of each is appropriate depends on the specific decision. For example, if you have pneumonia, it would be inappropriate for me as a doctor to say, "Would you like some antibiotics? Which one works best for you?" On the other hand, if we are discussing whether you should have an epidural in labor, it would also be inappropriate for me to say, "You need one" or "Do not get one" (there are exceptions to this, but those situations are rare).

One of the true arts in medicine is knowing when to be direct and make a recommendation, and when to hold back and let the patient direct the decision. As a patient, one of the ways to know you have a good doctor is when they find that right balance—you don't want a doctor who always tells you what to do and offers you no options, but you also don't want a doctor who won't ever give you their opinion.

So, my hope for this book is that it will better prepare you to have these types of conversations with your doctor, but also will give you a better insight into the medical side itself so you can have a greater sense of which decisions are best to make yourself and which decisions might make more sense to lean on the doctor for.

HOW SHOULD I USE THIS BOOK?

We designed this book to be read in two parts. The first part deals with preparation. This is intended to provide all readers a general framework for how you might approach a pregnancy with or after complications. We'll talk through what kind of information you want to collect about your own medical history, as well as some decision-making tools that may be useful in thinking about how you want to move forward.

The second part of the book is divided into condition-specific chapters. These are designed to be read as needed. In some cases, you may need multiple chapters. In others, only one. In each chapter case we talk through the data on recurrence and prevention and then offer a perspective from Nate on how to approach conversations with your providers about these issues.*

---

* There will be some overlap in the book across chapters; we've intended for you to be able to read the chapters you need.

Another option, of course, is to read all the chapters. Even if a specific complication is not relevant to you, the process we go through for thinking about the issue—and developing a framework for patients to think about it with family members and doctors—might speak to you in other areas of your journey through pregnancy, or health care in general.

We have tried hard to cover a large share of the major issues that arise in pregnancy, birth, and afterward. However, there will inevitably be conditions or circumstances we have missed. In these cases, we hope that going back through the first part of the book will give you a place to begin as you proceed in conversations with your own providers.

Although this book is written primarily with an eye to second pregnancies, you may find it helpful for some complications in a first pregnancy as well. If you are struggling with a condition like hyperemesis gravidarum, gestational diabetes, or growth restriction, for instance, the chapters on these topics will hopefully give you a starting point to discuss treatment and approaches with your provider.

Finally, a note that these issues are hard. They are hard to experience, hard to read about, hard to write about. So, while I hope this book helps, I also ask you to take care of yourself when you read. Take a break and have a cup of tea, or go for a walk. Nate and I will be here when you get back.

PART 1

Preparation

efore we get into conditions, this section starts with some general principles that will apply to virtually everyone reading this book. We'll talk through these ideas in the next three chapters.

First, prepare yourself. Engage with the question of a possible future pregnancy. Is this the right choice? Is now the right time? How can you know if you're ready?

Second, prepare your material. Get your medical records. Talk to your doctor about your last pregnancy. You are the best keeper of your own information, and having it at your fingertips will be helpful. This can—and, if possible, should—be done close to the first pregnancy. This is when your case will be most fresh in your mind, and in the mind of your provider. Even if you aren't sure about a future pregnancy, you may want to collect this information just in case.

Third, prepare your script. The first visit with a provider—either before another pregnancy, or once you're pregnant—is an opportunity to set expectations and make a plan. We want you to feel prepared for this conversation. This chapter should help you think about that script.

There is one more, very crucial, note. If a pregnancy didn't go the way you planned—*regardless of the outcome*—there can be a sense of loss. Of course this is the case with miscarriage or stillbirth. But it's also true for birth trauma, for preterm birth, for having a cesarean delivery if you anticipated a vaginal birth, or for any unexpected or difficult portion of the pregnancy and birth.

We naturally come into a first pregnancy with a set of expectations for pregnancy and birth. If your experience differs from those expectations, that can bring on grief. That sense of loss is commonly dismissed—"Well, you had a healthy baby! You don't have to worry about what happened before." This is, frankly, bullshit. Yes, experiences vary, and some people are able to accept what happened more easily than others. But you deserve to process in whatever way you need to.

So before you do any of the concrete steps in this book, get the support—therapy, writing, meditation, whatever works for you—that you need now.

~~~~~~~~~~

CHAPTER 1

Prepare Yourself

There are many technical things to do to prepare for another pregnancy after one that was complicated: collect medical records, decide about doctor changes, perhaps undergo additional testing. We'll talk about all of that in depth in the next chapter. Before any of this, though, you need to do perhaps the most important thing: prepare yourself emotionally.

So, what does that mean?

Very broadly, it means looking back on what happened before, trying to process it, and thinking deliberately about your steps going forward. It sounds straightforward in theory, yet it can be anything but.

What this means for you will depend tremendously on what happened. Complicated pregnancies take many forms, and both the medical and the emotional experience will inform what comes next.

What is obvious to most people is that your history will influence the medical choices in a later pregnancy. What may be less obvious but equally important is the recognition that the *life choices* you make may be affected by this history. More specifically: it may make sense to engage in detailed planning for a possible repeat of complications in a later pregnancy even if there is nothing to do medically.

Many of the people I spoke with for this book hadn't been encouraged to think about this step.

Consider one woman who suffered from hyperemesis gravidarum (severe nausea and vomiting):

• • •

One year after our son was born, we began the discussion of a second. We talked through the cost of child care, impacts to our careers (both were taking off), desired age gap between children, and the belief in our ability to handle two children. The discussion of my experience with HG never came up . . .

• • •

In this case, HG did return during her second pregnancy, and the experience was extremely challenging for the entire family. It is not clear that her choice to conceive again would have been impacted by this risk, but if they had grappled with it from the beginning, they would have been able to put more support in place. They could have had a more concrete plan for backup childcare. She could have had a conversation with her employer about how her team could have prepared to adapt if necessary. There are a variety of ways this might have made the experience at least somewhat easier than the previous.

One reason I think people avoid these questions is that we require acknowledgment of things we wish were not true. Acknowledging the fact that this debilitating pregnancy condition might return in a later pregnancy forces us to live with that uncomfortable reality—past, present, and future. In the moment, it's easier to live with the hope that it won't happen again. Of course, doing so may leave us unprepared. Hard as this is, I urge you not to skip this ultimately healing step.

A second problem is that it can be hard to know how to approach what comes next. Sometimes, it's hard to even know what you're trying to think about or prepare for. Is your key question whether to have another child? Is it how to prepare for that? Is it both? The issues raised by complicated pregnancies are large and varied, and it can be difficult to know where to start. Process can help.

When the questions are uncertain and hard, it is easy for your experience to drag on without resolution. It is almost impossible to know if you are making the right decision, which makes it tempting to make no decision at all. Ultimately, you'll be better prepared for whatever decision you make, though, if you commit to making it deliberately.

In my book *The Family Firm*, I talk through a structured process—the Four Fs—to approach big decisions. I think this provides a useful starting point in deciding whether to try getting pregnant again and for many of the other decisions we'll address in this book.

STEP 1: FRAME THE QUESTION

You cannot make plans or prepare without clarifying what you are trying to decide or to accomplish. The first step, then, is to frame the question.

After a complicated pregnancy, for many, the question is simply whether to try for another child. This is an example of a question where it is very important to be explicit about alternatives. It's easy to state this question as "Should we try for another pregnancy or not?" That framing isn't explicit enough about what "or not" means. There are other ways to grow a family—adoption, surrogacy—that may be a possibility for some people. "Or not" does not allow for the nuances of timing. Are you really asking whether you should have another pregnancy now or *never*? Or is it now versus waiting a year, or two, or waiting *x* amount of time and then reconsidering at that point?

For other people, the choice to have another pregnancy may be an obvious one, and the question may be about timing. After a miscarriage, for example, people often struggle with the question of whether to try again right away or to wait. The question "Should we try again now?" might be better framed as "Should we try again now or revisit the timing in three months?" Because this framing is explicit about the choice—it's not "now or never" but "now or in the relatively near future"—it may make it easier to recognize the need to wait.

Or the appropriate question may be about support. "What support systems should we have in place before trying again? Should we invite my mother to live with us in the event that the pregnancy is complicated?"

This question framing is an opportunity to clarify priorities. Are all family members committed to having more children? And if so, are you emotionally ready to consider trying again, especially after loss? It is reasonable—common—for people to differ on these questions, even people who are building a life together. They are often not questions we confront when we first start trying for a family. This moment is an opportunity to confront them, to figure out what decision we need to make about going forward.

STEP 2: FACT FIND

Get all the information you can in order to be prepared for whatever may come next.

For example, imagine your first pregnancy was complicated by preeclampsia at 25 weeks, followed by seven weeks of in-hospital bed rest and then six weeks in the NICU with your baby. When considering another pregnancy, your first question will probably be how likely this is to happen again. Should you expect a repeat experience? You'll probably also ask what might be done to reduce the risk of recurrence or to improve the outcome. It isn't possible to prevent many of the complications we discuss throughout the book, but knowing the possible risks allows you and your provider to treat the condition better and have a better outcome.

When considering another pregnancy you should also take into account how your family would approach the situation. What supports could you have in place to take care of your existing child if you had to be hospitalized again? If you are working, what preparations might you make professionally? Of course, we can vehemently hope that the condition will not recur, in which case these questions would have been unnecessary. But confronting how you would deal with these complications again should be a part of both preparing and, possibly, of making your decision about moving forward.

This step may take some time; in many cases, it will make sense to speak with your medical provider. In the particular case above, you might raise the question of alternatives to bed rest. This is an opportunity to talk about whether that's something that the provider would insist on if it happened again, or whether there would be options that might be a better fit for your family.

The goal of this step is to get the information you need—all of it—to make the decision you're facing, whatever it is.

STEPS 3 AND 4:
FINAL DECISION AND FOLLOW-UP

Having asked a specific question and collected the information you need, you can come together to make a final decision.

We've intentionally left space for deliberate follow-up in some of these situations. Waiting is one possible decision. Rather than trying to conceive immediately, you may choose to wait and see how things look in three months (or six months, or a year). If you explicitly decide to wait, you can then also set a time when you'll revisit the decision.

The two approaches—committing to a decision or committing to a follow-up time, if appropriate—may help some people move forward. If you've had two miscarriages in rapid succession and the past months have been a devastating period of back-to-back losses, it may help to say, simply, "We are not going to think about this for another six months." Sometimes self-care is the only, and best, possible goal.

CHAPTER 2

Prepare Your Materials

The last chapter talked about the process of deciding whether to embark on a second pregnancy, and in what way. If you do decide on another pregnancy, you'll face more practical questions. This chapter is about the first steps in that practical stage: collecting the information you'll need to have the most productive conversations with your provider.

Remember that you are the keeper of your information, and you (and your partner) are your own best advocate. Your provider is an amazing, crucial resource, but you ultimately may need to be the one who takes ownership of your own experience and tracks your records and history.

Ground yourself in the necessity of accuracy and honesty, both for yourself and for your provider. We have a tendency to downplay our own experiences—the pain, the nausea, the discomfort "wasn't that bad." But you'll be better positioned for success if you can be open about your experiences and how they felt to you.

STEP 1: CHOOSE YOUR PROVIDER

Many people keep the same provider across pregnancies. However, there are cases in which it makes sense to switch, and this may be more true for those with complicated past pregnancies. It therefore makes sense to at least consider this possibility.

There are two possible reasons you might want to switch providers. The most obvious one is that you didn't like your doctor or midwife. It can be hard to talk about, but sometimes the doctor-patient relationship just isn't working. It should be possible to acknowledge this without layering on any value judgment. The doctor could be great, but not great *for you*. Pregnancy and childbirth are significant medical and personal experiences, and you deserve to feel comfortable, whatever that means to you. If the doctor-patient relationship didn't work for you, that is a good reason to switch. Similarly, you may prefer a larger practice with many options of providers, or you may prefer a smaller practice with only one or two providers. There are upsides and downsides to both types of practices, and your preference matters.

The second reason you might switch is if you need or want a provider with a different specialty. In the US, most babies are delivered by physicians who are specialists in obstetrics and gynecology (OB-GYNs). OB-GYNs practice at hospitals (or, in some rare cases, at birthing centers) and are trained in both vaginal and cesarean deliveries. For most women, this is the default provider specialty. Other physicians who might provide prenatal care and delivery are specialists in family practice.

Each year, about 8 percent of infants in the US are delivered by midwives. A midwife can be an excellent option if your pregnancy is low risk, but this is often not the best option if there are particular risk factors. If you used a midwife in a first pregnancy and had certain complications, it might make sense to switch to an OB-GYN.

Sometimes, based on what happened in your previous pregnancy or your current risk factors, you may want to consider consulting with, or switching to, a maternal-fetal medicine specialist (MFM). MFMs are OB-GYNs who have done three additional years of subspecialty training in high-risk pregnancies and fetal diagnosis, such as ultrasound, chorionic villus sampling (CVS), amniocentesis, and fetal blood sampling. Some MFMs continue to practice OB-GYN as well, doing prenatal care and deliveries, while others work only as consultants, seeing you in addition to your own OB-GYN either once or on an ongoing basis, based on the circumstances. Colloquially, they are sometimes called high-risk OB-GYNs or perinatologists (not to be confused with neonatologists, who take care of newborn babies).

(For example, Nate is an MFM who continues to do prenatal care and deliveries in addition to consultations and ultrasound, but he has partners who are MFMs and only do consultations and ultrasound. Nate apparently enjoys being up late at night . . .)

In the United States, the availability of MFMs differs regionally. In some areas, there are many MFMs practicing, including those who do deliveries, and in other areas there may be fewer MFMs, and none who do deliveries. If you are considering transferring care to an MFM, you need to do some research and locate MFMs near you, if any, and find out if they do prenatal care and deliveries (usually this information is listed on their website, or you can just call the office and ask). It is important to note that an MFM certification does not specifically indicate that the doctor is "better" at deliveries. The MFM distinction is mostly related to managing a high-risk *pregnancy*, not a delivery. If you have a high-risk pregnancy, there is usually nothing wrong with consulting with an MFM and being delivered by an OB-GYN. It may be more convenient to have all your care with one doctor, or one practice, but it is not necessarily better. Therefore, if all that is available to you is consultation with an MFM, and not delivery, it will still have a meaningful impact.

Having a consultation with an MFM should be an option for everyone, especially with the availability of telehealth and virtual visits. For most MFM consultations, there is no examination required; a conversation over a videoconference platform is a great way to have the initial consultation. For many pregnancies, ultrasounds are recommended for follow-up, so there will need to be some in-person visits, but the MFM should be able to provide information on which visits require ultrasounds, and where they should take place.

Typically, the increased frequency of ultrasounds would be to assess the growth, health, and development of the fetus, or to screen for the risk of preterm birth with a transvaginal measurement of the length of your cervix. The MFM should also be able to determine whether you need further MFM follow-up at routine intervals or only if certain complications arise. This will differ for each individual circumstance. It is possible you may need a referral from your OB-GYN or midwife to see an MFM for a consultation, but that differs across practices and insurances.

While we are on this topic, a short note on costs and insurance. One could easily write a whole book about the challenges of our health care system, and many have. But for our purposes here, you should be aware that some of the treatments discussed in this book, and the evaluations, can be expensive. Generally speaking, these will be covered by insurance if you have it. There may be cases in which there are a surprising number of hoops to jump through to get the treatment you need, although usually your provider can help you figure out these challenges.

Ultimately, choosing a provider—as with the first time around—should be about finding someone you are comfortable with who will serve your needs.

STEP 2: COLLECT YOUR DATA

As will be clear in much of this book, every complicated pregnancy is complicated in its own way. We can talk about some general numbers, but your experience is unique. The details of that experience are important for understanding possible steps in a later pregnancy. Especially if you switch providers, but even if not, having a complete sense of your own history is central.

As we noted at the start of this section, getting this history as close as possible to the time of your first pregnancy will be helpful. Even though you may have been through an arduous ordeal, we encourage you to ask questions. That information will empower any future attempt at pregnancy you make. It may be possible to have this conversation later, if it does not happen at the time.

Key questions to ask your providers include:

1. Are you able to explain in simple terms what happened to me and, if you know, why it happened to me?
2. What important tests did I have and what did they reveal? Were any of them abnormal?

3. What treatments did I receive? Which ones worked and which ones didn't?

4. Was I seen by other specialists? If so, what did they contribute?

5. What are the facts I need to know if I were to try to explain this accurately to another doctor?

6. Is there anything I need to do or know prior to another pregnancy?

7. Is there anything you would recommend I do differently, or a treatment I should receive, in a future pregnancy?

(You can ask the same questions about your baby, if those are relevant to your specific situation.)

In addition, getting copies of your pertinent medical records is a very good idea. Since electronic medical records are (sadly) hundreds or even thousands of pages long, here is a list of the (typically) most important records:

1. A summary of what happened, in your own words, as detailed as possible. Do not assume you will remember these details forever. Write them down!

2. A summary of what happened, written by your provider. This might be in a "pregnancy history" in your prenatal chart or a "discharge summary" if you were in a hospital. If you don't think there is a written summary available, you can ask your provider to write one for you.

3. If you had a cesarean delivery, or any other operation in pregnancy or after delivery, a copy of the "operative report" (aka the "op note"). This is a detailed description written by the surgeon of what they did during the operation, and why.

4. A copy of your "delivery summary." These take different forms, but pretty much all electronic medical records have a summary of the delivery, such as birth time, Apgar scores, blood loss, and a description by the delivering provider of what happened.

5. The results from all blood tests, imaging (ultrasound, CT scan, etc.), pathology (placenta, biopsies), and genetic testing.

6. Copies of any consultations done by other specialists. Nearly always, the specialist will write a report summarizing their findings and impressions.

This list is not comprehensive, but it's a great way to ensure that you have the most important information available to you and your future doctors. Although you may need to sign a release form and you may need to pay a nominal fee to have records printed or copied, by federal law the records are yours, not the doctor's or hospital's, and you are absolutely entitled to copies of anything and everything you request. Note: Sometimes the hospital or doctor's office will tell you that they need to send the records to another provider, but that is not correct. You are absolutely entitled to receive a copy of the records yourself.

STEP 3: POSSIBLE ADDITIONAL TESTING

Depending on the particular complication you had, there are a number of additional tests that your provider might recommend. These are discussed in more detail in the context of each condition. Regardless of your complication, however, it may make sense to consider genetic carrier screening. This screening may be possible to organize before any doctor's visit so that you have the information to begin discussions.

Genetic carrier screening is a blood test that checks if you are a carrier for any genetic conditions that can be passed on to your children. As a review from high school biology class, humans have 46 chromosomes in each cell, arranged as 23 pairs (numbered 1 through 22, with the 23rd being the X or Y chromosome). You get one set of 23 chromosomes from your father and one set of 23 chromosomes from your mother. An autosomal recessive condition is one that is caused by a genetic mutation but that manifests as a disease only if you have the mutation on *both* copies of that chromosome. If you have one mutated and one normal chromosome, you are perfectly fine, but you are a carrier.

If two carriers have a child together, there is a 25 percent chance that the child will have the full disease. Here's how that works:

A = normal gene
a = mutated gene

AA = healthy, noncarrier
Aa = healthy, carrier
aa = disease

If two carriers (Aa and Aa) conceive a child together:

	A	a
A	AA (heathy, noncarrier), 25%	Aa (healthy, carrier), 25%
a	Aa (healthy, carrier), 25%	aa (disease), 25%

Twenty-five percent will have the disease.

Seventy-five percent will be healthy (broken down as 50 percent healthy carriers and 25 percent healthy noncarriers).

A well-known example of an autosomal recessive disease is Tay-Sachs, a devastating neurological condition for which the life expectancy is only a few years. Individuals with one copy of the genetic mutation are unaffected; those with two will have the disease.

There are hundreds of autosomal genetic conditions that can be carried and passed on in this manner, and if you aren't screened for them, you would have no way of knowing you are a carrier. Given the volume of conditions, there is about a 70 percent chance you carry at least one condition, but fortunately only about a 2 to 5 percent chance you and your partner are carriers for the same condition, which is the only situation that is potentially an issue. It is important to note that many autosomal recessive conditions are not very serious, but it may still be good to be aware of them.

This testing can be done in pregnancy, but it is better done prior to pregnancy, since if you find out you are both carriers of the same condition, you have more options, including doing IVF to test the embryos for the condition (PGT, or preimplantation genetic testing) and then only use embryos without the disease.

This is also the kind of testing that needs to be updated because over the past twenty years, our knowledge of genetic disease causes has expanded exponentially as we discover more conditions or more mutations of known conditions. The panels, which initially tested for five conditions, now cover over five hundred, so if you did a screening for your first pregnancy, it would make sense to check if the screening panel has been expanded before your next pregnancy. Depending on where you live and, unfortunately, the quality of your insurance, you may have access to more or less of these tests. It is worth asking your provider what they recommend and also what they offer if you want to do more than their standard approach.

~~~

CHAPTER 3

Prepare Your Script

There is often a very large gap between the medical knowledge you can have as a patient—even as a very well-informed patient—and what your doctor knows based on their training and experience.

One of the primary goals of this book is to build a bridge over the knowledge gap, at least a bit. When we talk about individual conditions in the later sections of this book, I'll try to give a sense of the data so you have the background. Nate will talk through the perspective your doctor may be bringing to the conversation.

This information will help. But what will also help is bringing structure to the appointment. In this chapter, we'll outline a bit of a script for how to approach *any* of these conversations.

Our suggestion, based on Nate's experience, is to write a script aimed at answering four key questions:

1. What happened?
2. Why did it happen to me?

3. Is it going to happen to me again?

4. What can be done to prevent it from happening again (or to lessen the severity)?

QUESTION 1: WHAT HAPPENED?

This question may seem obvious—in some broad sense, you know what happened. The goal of this first part of the script is to get to the details. In many cases, the details of your history are going to be key to understanding solutions.

For example, consider someone whose last pregnancy was delivered at 37 weeks with preeclampsia. There are numerous reasons why this would occur, and the implications for the future often depend on exactly what happened. In this type of case, Nate would ask (or would review) a whole series of questions:

- Was the preeclampsia diagnosed before, during, or after labor?
- What were the symptoms or test results that led to the diagnosis?
- Did you go into labor on your own, or did something happen that caused a doctor to recommend delivery?
- Was there bleeding, and, if so, was it before or during labor?
- Did you get any medications before or after birth to lower your blood pressure?
- Did you get intravenous magnesium before labor, during labor, after delivery, or some combination of those?
- Did you have abnormal blood tests?
- When was the most recent ultrasound before you delivered, and what did it show?

- Was the placenta examined after birth by a pathologist?
- How big was your baby at birth?
- How long did you need to stay in the hospital after birth?
- Did you need to go home from the hospital on blood-pressure medications?
- How long did it take for your blood pressure to get better?

Going through a detailed set of questions like this provides a necessary and nuanced picture of the particular case. Most conditions come in many varieties, with possibly different approaches.

For this part of the conversation, your medical records and your recollections are likely to be crucial. Starting the appointment with these on hand will enable you and your provider to get the most out of this part of the conversation.

QUESTION 2: WHY DID IT HAPPEN TO ME?

This is a complicated question, and of course one way to read it is, "What did I do to deserve this?" or "Was this my fault?"

It is extremely common to grapple with these questions. For many people, therapy can be hugely helpful in working through these feelings.

But, from the standpoint of looking forward, the question of fault is not relevant. It's not just that, in nearly all cases, complications aren't about fault. It's that even if they were, our goal moving forward is to use the tools we have to reduce the risk that this happens again.

With that lens, when we ask "Why did this happen to me?," what we mean is much more practical: "Did I have an increased risk for this complication going *into* the last pregnancy?" More specifically, we want to try to establish whether it seems like the prior complication was predictable based on known factors.

For example, if someone had a preterm birth, we might ask whether she was carrying twins or whether preterm birth runs in her family. If she had twins in the last pregnancy, then it is very likely that the preterm birth was because of the multiple gestation; the risk in a later pregnancy with a singleton gestation isn't necessarily elevated. In contrast, if preterm birth runs in her family, this could suggest a systematically increased risk.

Most risk factors for complications are what we refer to as *non-modifiable* (i.e., out of your control)—for example, age, family history, and genetics. Some risk factors are *potentially modifiable*. For example, getting pregnant through IVF increases the risk of some complications. This is potentially modifiable since, in principle, you could get pregnant in another way. But this may be practically useless advice since for most couples using IVF there isn't an alternative. Smoking and body weight are *modifiable* risk factors for many conditions, but as anyone who is a smoker or has ever tried to lose weight knows, it's not so easy to do.

The goal in addressing this "why" question is to learn which, if any, risk factors were present that might help explain the complication. If it's possible to identify these (and, to be clear, many complications occur with no risk factors), we can then ask whether any of these risk factors are modifiable in the next pregnancy.

QUESTION 3:
IS IT GOING TO HAPPEN TO ME AGAIN?

This is the crux of the conversation, and it's the hardest question. It's usually also one without a precise answer. Our lives would be a lot easier if we could answer this question definitively. If it were possible to divide people into those who are going to have the complication again and those who are not, we could provide appropriate high-risk care to those who would have it again and standard low-risk care to those who would not.

For now, we do not have a crystal ball for this. It may be that one day, with advances in precision medicine, we can come closer. For now, the best we can do is *percentages*.

Throughout this book, we'll look at data on risk of recurrence for various conditions. Based (often) on large datasets, we'll be able to make claims like, "On average, 25 to 50 percent of women who had preeclampsia in one pregnancy will have it in a later pregnancy." These numbers can be useful as a benchmark, but they are challenging in at least two ways.

First, your individual risk is likely to vary significantly based on your circumstances. To continue with the preeclampsia example, for someone who had preeclampsia with onset at 28 weeks and severe symptoms, their risk of recurrence is high—probably higher than 50 percent. For someone who had onset at 39 weeks, with only limited symptoms, the recurrence risk is much lower (and severe recurrence is even less likely).

Second, the exact percentage frequently doesn't matter, or doesn't matter precisely. Think about a recurrence risk of 20 percent versus

40 percent. These numbers are different. But most humans—even those of us who work with probabilities for a living—have a hard time really understanding these differences in a way that aids in decision making. There *are* differences that we can understand. Most people are able to conceptualize that a 5 percent probability of recurrence and a 75 percent probability are different, and that difference is enough that it could be helpful in decision making. A 20 percent probability of recurrence versus 40 percent is not like that.

This leads to one possibly helpful way to conceptualize recurrence risks, which is categorization. Nate often uses categories in addition to a precise number.

1. Very unlikely to recur (we try to quantify that number as less than 10 percent, less than 5 percent, and less than 1 percent).
2. Increased risk compared with someone else, but still could go either way. Based on the particular complication, this is usually in the 20 to 50 percent range.
3. Expect it to happen, and if it doesn't, that's fortunate. This is something greater than 50 percent.

Getting more precise than that is rarely helpful.

A third reason why assessing recurrence risks can be unhelpful is that, for some outcomes, it isn't all or none (yes or no). For example, if someone had hyperemesis gravidarum that was so severe that she needed to be hospitalized for three months in her pregnancy, she may not care if her next pregnancy technically qualifies as HG or not (there are criteria). It may matter more to her if we can manage it to a state of simply being *less* miserable and where she's not in the hospital. So even if her chance of recurrence is over 50 percent, it's more important if we have options that could make her *experience* of the complication different.

In this part of the conversation, then, the goal should be to use the first part of the discussion to get to a range of possibilities. Should you think of your prior experience as more or less uninformative? Or should we plan with the expectation that this is likely to happen, in some form, again?

QUESTION 4: WHAT CAN BE DONE TO PREVENT IT FROM HAPPENING AGAIN (OR TO LESSEN THE SEVERITY)?

This final step in the conversation is about two things. First, is it possible to change the risk of recurrence with particular interventions? Second, can we improve the treatment situation if the condition does occur again?

For example, if you had preeclampsia in your first pregnancy and therefore have an increased risk of it in your second pregnancy, both of these strategies apply. We can try to lower the risk with, for example, low-dose aspirin during pregnancy. But even if our interventions do not completely prevent preeclampsia, it is possible they may delay the onset or decrease the severity. Think about this in parallel to the COVID or flu vaccine. Neither vaccine eliminates your risk of getting the virus, but both dramatically decrease the severity if you do get it. Similarly, here we are often looking for interventions that would make things better.

Some of these interventions are about reducing the chance of a condition or delaying onset. Others are about better preparing for what you do if it does happen. When we talk about postpartum mental health challenges, for example, the risk of recurrence is very high. But, knowing this, we can be prepared to treat this quickly when it arises.

SUMMARY

Working from this script can go a long way toward making your first provider conversation as useful as possible. You're not going to get all the answers in one visit, and some of what may come out of the discussion is a plan to collect more information. But now you at least have a starting point.

PART 2

Complications

With the general background above, we are going to turn now to individual conditions. As I noted in the introduction, you may end up reading only one, or a couple, of these chapters. Our goal is for each of them to be self-contained, so you can read what you need.

However, there are a few issues I want to address here at the top because they are relevant for many or most of the following chapters. First, a quick primer on data. Second, a brief discussion of the role of race (with more resources for follow-up). Third, a comment on how the changing landscape of reproductive rights impacts the issues in the book.

A PRIMER ON DATA

In discussing individual conditions, we'll come back again and again to two key questions in the data.

First, what is the recurrence risk? If something happened before, what is the chance it will happen again?

Second, how can I prevent it? What *modifiable* treatments could make a difference?

The first of these questions is really about *prediction*. The second is about *causal inference*.

The distinction matters. To see why prediction and causal inference are different, it's useful to think about a different context. Imagine you're working in online advertising. Your goal is to show ads for shampoo to people who are most likely to click on them. You have some information about people—which other websites they visit, what items they've purchased in the past, etc. To be successful in your goal, you should use all the information you have about people to predict whether they'll click on your shampoo ad. Once you've got a good predictive model, you can use that to target ads.

What is important to note is that in this setting, you do not care *why* your prediction works well. Let's say you find that people who purchase their paper towels in twelve-packs are more likely to click on ads for shampoo than people who purchase paper towels in packs of six. From your standpoint, that is really valuable information for ad targeting. But it actually doesn't matter much to you *why* this correlation is there. You just care that it is predictive.

When we ask about the risk of recurrence, we are effectively asking whether having had a condition before is predictive of having it again, and to what extent. We may be less interested in *why* it is predictive—there are many reasons why a condition might repeat itself. What matters is the chance that it does.

These kinds of prediction problems are very amenable to big-data analysis because they can be answered with passively collected data. Many countries, especially in Europe, have extensive anonymized records in which people can be linked across their pregnancies. With this type of data you can ask, for example, whether women who had preeclampsia in a first pregnancy are more likely to have it again in a second, and how much more likely. In some cases there is also information on what other characteristics predict recurrence, and where they modify the impacts of the previous condition.

What about causal inference? Let's return to our shampoo ads. We talked about predicting who would click based on what you know about them. You also might want to ask whether some ads perform better than others. Maybe you have two possible taglines—"Sleek and Shiny" or "Soft and Silky." In order to decide between them, you'd run an experiment.

This is pretty easy when you're doing online advertising. You run both ads online and randomize who sees which one (this is sometimes called A/B testing). Because you've chosen at random who sees which ad, if you see people click more on one ad than the other, you can be confident that it is a causal effect. In this case, you *do* care about the effect being causal, because you want to choose which ad to push out to everyone. And to make that decision, you want to be confident that it is the ad choice that is driving the clicks.

This is analogous to the second question: Can I prevent this? When we evaluate whether a particular treatment lowers the risk of complications, we are asking a causal question. If we did this treatment with someone at risk, would their likelihood of having the condition recur be lower? The best way to answer these questions—really, the only reliable way—is with a randomized controlled trial in which you give the treatment to a randomly chosen subset of a group and not to the rest. You compare their outcomes, and if the treated group had better outcomes, that's the conclusion.

This type of question is not easily answered with the big registry-based datasets that we can use for prediction. Even if there is variation in treatments used within those datasets, if that variation is not explicitly random, we cannot draw causal conclusions.

To be concrete, we can return to the shampoo ad example. Imagine we have a large dataset with household purchases, and we observe, again, that people who purchase large packs of paper towels are more likely to buy shampoo. Although it might be tempting to conclude that there is something causal here—that purchasing a lot of towels somehow causes you to need more frequent hair washing—that wouldn't be supported by the data. It's much more likely that other factors would drive this correlation. To draw meaningful causal conclusions, we need a randomized trial.

Ultimately, in both shampoo and pregnancy, the prediction question is much easier to answer because it's more amenable to data that is easier to access.

However, even the question of recurrence is often not straightforward. For one thing, there may be significant *heterogeneity* across people or groups. Much of our data comes from Europe, or from European populations. The extent to which race or ethnicity impacts recurrence risks may be hard to capture.

But arguably more important, there is uncertainty. In nearly every case—every complication—there are likely to be many contributing factors. No one variable will explain all cases, and no one treatment will eliminate all problems. There are virtually no complications for which there is 100 percent recurrence, or 0 percent recurrence. At least some people who had any complication in a prior pregnancy will not have it again, and some people will have it again.

When we look at studies of interventions, we often see something like this:

Four hundred women with a prior spontaneous preterm birth were randomly divided into two groups. Group 1 received intervention X, and group 2 received a placebo or no intervention. We examined the likelihood of recurrent preterm birth in the two groups:

> Group 1 (received intervention X): 20 percent delivered preterm
>
> Group 2 (did not receive intervention X): 40 percent delivered preterm

Therefore, intervention X is effective in reducing the risk of recurrent preterm birth.

While this study does in fact suggest that intervention X is effective in reducing the risk of recurrent preterm birth, there is much more richness in the data.

First, the group that got the intervention still had a 20 percent risk of preterm birth (the baseline risk in the population is about 10 percent, so this group still has twice the typical risk), meaning the intervention didn't work for everyone. This makes sense when we understand that there are different reasons you might deliver preterm, and a particular intervention might target only one or two of them.

Second, in the group that did not get any intervention, only 40 percent delivered preterm, meaning 60 percent delivered at term without any intervention at all. This also makes sense when we understand that many of the reasons you might deliver preterm are not going to happen again in the next pregnancy, because they happened by chance and not due to some inherent predisposition that you have.

Much of the work of this book will be in these questions of prediction and causal inference. I'll try to work through the factors that predict recurrence and, when we have it, discuss the treatments that we might have causal data for. Throughout, it will be important to keep this last point in mind: We'll deal in probabilities, risks, and improvements as a share of baseline. We will not deal in certainties. This is part of what makes these issues so complicated to work through—comparing risks is hard, and we do not like to live with uncertainty. But we must.

THE ROLE OF RACE

My goal in this book is to provide data on recurrence and treatment options that apply to all patients. In many cases, the treatments that work for preventing recurrence are not specific to race or ethnicity. Often, our best data on treatment comes from samples that are at least broadly representative in terms of racial groups.

However, the risk of the pregnancy complications we discuss here vary significantly by race in the US. In particular, Black women in the US have a much higher risk of pregnancy complications, including very serious ones, than women from other racial groups. The most extreme is the difference in maternal mortality. In 2021, the maternal mortality rate for Black women was 2.3 times as high as either Hispanic women or non-Hispanic white women.[1] Black women are at especially high risk for cardiovascular-related complications—preeclampsia, cardiomyopathy, stroke.

The reasons for these differences are complex. Differences in resources and underlying health surely play some role. However, neither differences in income nor a simple health metric like obesity seem to explain these differences. In the case of income, research has shown that maternal and infant health for Black mothers at the very top of the income distribution is worse than that for white mothers who are at the bottom.[2] As Dr. Joia Crear-Perry has said: "Black women cannot buy or educate their way out of dying at three to four times the rate of white mothers. Maternal mortality rates persist regardless of our class or education status."[3]

Researchers in this space have pointed to systemic racism as a driver of these differences. Research by Dr. Arline Geronimus on "weathering" has highlighted the impact of the stress of systemic racism on health outcomes.

In a similar vein, writing in *ParentData*, Dr. Quantrilla Ard argues:

> Consider this: there is literature citing the experience of Black birthing people who have immigrated to the United States as observed in birth weight. Low birth weight is a critical indicator of infant mortality. Foreign-born Black women have birth weights similar to US white women. However, birth weight declines significantly as generations of Black birthing people assimilate to the United States. There is something unique to the experience of being born Black in America that is disparately creating an environment of reproductive harm and disadvantage and killing Black birthing people and their babies. It is racism and the lived experience of racism, not race, that drives maternal and infant mortality rates for Black birthing people and their infants in the United States.[4]

Understanding what should be done to achieve health equity is an extremely important task for both research and policy. It is beyond the scope of this book to address these issues in detail, but there are many important scholars and authors who are doing this work, and in the appendix we have links to a number of books—*Weathering, Under the*

Skin, Thick, The Black Agenda—devoted to a focused engagement with these issues.

For Black readers, I hope that the data here will help you navigate provider conversations, just as I hope it will for everyone reading this book. I'd also direct you to work by Erica Chidi, the author of *Nurture*, who has done specific writing on navigating the landscape of pregnancy care as a Black woman. The resource section at the end of the book includes further recommendations.

CHANGING LANDSCAPE OF REPRODUCTIVE RIGHTS

In 2022, the Supreme Court's decision on *Dobbs v. Jackson Women's Health Organization* overturned the 1973 *Roe v. Wade* decision, which legalized abortion nationally. As a result, in many states abortion has been restricted or completely curtailed.

Abortion care overlaps with miscarriage care in many cases; the surgical procedure following a first- or second-trimester miscarriage is the same as the surgical procedure for an abortion in those time frames. While the decision in Dobbs does not directly curtail a doctor's ability to perform these procedures following a miscarriage, it may affect the amount of experience they have doing so, thereby limiting people's access to providers capable of safely performing those procedures.

In some cases we cover—like severe, early preeclampsia—the health of a fetus and the life of the mother may be at odds. Restrictions on abortion rights generally make exceptions for the life of the mother, but the details are often vague and vary greatly from state to state, and medical professionals may be unsure about what approaches are allowed under the law.

Frankly, this is scary, especially if you are at higher risk for complications in pregnancy. The best we can offer in this book is that you should have a conversation early on with your provider about what your options might be, and what resources are available, if necessary. Of particular note, the landscape of abortion rights differs greatly across states. Knowing the options in your own state, and possibly in those around you, may be the best way to prepare.

First-Trimester
Complications

CHAPTER 4

Hyperemesis Gravidarum

DEFINITION: Persistent severe vomiting leading to
weight loss and dehydration, as a condition
occurring during pregnancy

OVERALL PREVALENCE: 1 to 2 percent of all pregnancies

RECURRENCE RISK GROUP: Intermediate (10 to 50 percent)

Hyperemesis gravidarum (HG) is a condition characterized by debilitating nausea and vomiting during pregnancy. Technically, it is defined as severe vomiting leading to weight loss and dehydration. HG varies significantly across patients, but can be extremely serious. People with HG will need supportive care to make sure they stay sufficiently hydrated and nourished and, in some cases, hospitalization to manage these issues.

As background: About 50 percent of pregnant people have nausea and possibly some vomiting in the first trimester, but HG is not that. HG affects 1 to 2 percent of pregnancies, and it is unfortunately very difficult to manage, as it can almost never be "cured"; rather, patients must wait for it to resolve or wait for delivery. For some people, the symptoms are so severe that they choose to terminate an otherwise highly desired pregnancy because they are suffering so greatly. There are a number of possible treatments, and sometimes they provide relief, but they rarely make HG go away.

The medical literature is not definitive in delineating when nausea or vomiting transitions from being just a normal part of pregnancy to HG. There are different criteria used, but in its most basic sense, HG is when the nausea and vomiting are so severe that they prevent someone from getting the nutrition and water they need to be healthy. Signs include weight loss, significant loss of energy, signs of dehydration (weakness and decreased urine production, as well as very dark and concentrated urine), and certain blood test abnormalities. Left untreated, HG can cause serious short- and long-term consequences to the pregnant person, and can even be life-threatening. The only good news here is that HG does not tend to have an adverse effect on the fetus.

Unfortunately, we do not have a great understanding of why some people have HG and others don't; why one person can have HG in one pregnancy and not have it in another one; why it sometimes persists through delivery and other times resolves on its own, and when it does resolve on its own, why it resolves at one point in pregnancy versus another. We can assume genetic factors are at play but also believe that other health or environmental factors matter.

Whatever the cause, HG can be an incredibly isolating experience, and one in which many patients simply feel dismissed or discounted.

Because so many people *have* had the mild or moderate nausea experience, they can unintentionally be callous. One woman with this condition talked candidly about the feeling of being dismissed—the feeling that other people thought she was, effectively, just overreacting.

• • •

The feedback I got from friends and even my in-laws was, "Oh, so-and-so also threw up a bunch; you'll be fine." A real peak was getting a text saying, "Oh, I was nauseous too; try the ginger gummies from Whole Foods." (I was in the hospital getting fluids when I got that text.)

• • •

Nate recalls one patient of his who desperately wanted a large family, but every pregnancy was complicated by HG. Essentially, the first three to four months of her pregnancies she had to stay home in bed. Nate's team was able to treat her effectively enough that she remained out of the hospital and healthy (which was a win), but they were never able to do better than that. So, every time she became pregnant she had some joy, but it was overtaken by profound misery over what she knew lay ahead. The thing that bothered her most was not her symptoms but rather the judgment of family and friends. The messaging she heard was: If you are so miserable when you are pregnant, don't have more kids. And if you do choose to get pregnant, don't be so miserable.

Many women who had HG expressed deep uncertainty and fear about later pregnancies.

• • •

I loathed the idea of being pregnant again, and now that we have two healthy children, we are absolutely not having any more.

We always knew we wanted two kids, but I was still afraid of getting sick again. We got pregnant again easily and I got sick earlier this time, and I was terrified and crying and telling my husband "I don't think I can do this" and briefly considered terminating.

• • •

That second person quoted here did not terminate their pregnancy, but the fear in that comment is visceral.

The data in the following section may not initially inspire confidence. Recurrence is fairly likely. However, being aware of the possibility can improve management and treatment.

WHAT THE DATA SAYS: RECURRENCE AND TREATMENT

Recurrence

In summary reports in the medical literature on the recurrence rates for HG, the estimated range is alarmingly broad. One systematic review puts the recurrence rate between 15 and 81 percent.[1] That range is so large as to be, effectively, useless. If this risk matters for your decisions, it's hard to imagine that you'd make the same ones if the risk is 1 in 7 versus 9 in 10. We discussed in the first part of this book the reality that it's difficult to distinguish small probability differences. However, 15 and 81 percent are *big* differences.

Fortunately, in this case a more fine-grained analysis of the data allows a much smaller range.

The largest studies of the condition come from Scandinavia. In Norway, one paper analyzed data from a registry of pregnant women who gave birth between 1967 and 1998.[2] There are close to 550,000 women in the registry, of whom researchers identified 4,700 with HG in their first pregnancy. Among these, 15.2 percent of them had recurrence in their second pregnancy (versus 0.7 percent during a second pregnancy for those who did not have it in their first).

A second paper, from Finland, takes a similar approach.[3] In it, researchers took into account all deliveries in Finland from 2004 to 2011. They identified 1,835 first pregnancies that included an HG diagnosis; these were followed by 2,267 subsequent pregnancies. The data showed that recurrence occurred in 24 percent of the subsequent pregnancies.

These papers highlight any HG diagnosis, not the severity. To better understand that dimension, we can look at a study from the UK that includes more than 8 million pregnancies and found that women who had HG in a prior pregnancy had about a 10 percent chance of being hospitalized for HG in a current pregnancy. This contrasts to only 2 percent for those without an HG diagnosis in a prior pregnancy.[4]

Twenty-four percent and 10 percent are much closer to 15 percent than 81 percent, leaving us with the question: Where does the 81 percent come from? The answer is one small study of fifty-seven women who had HG in their first pregnancy and completed an online survey about it in their second.[5] In this case, 81 percent reported a second diagnosis.

From a research standpoint, we would always favor a study that includes the entire population of Norway over a sample of fifty-seven people who chose to participate in an online survey. It's easy to see why the selection process for that type of online survey could produce overestimates of the recurrence risk.

However, there is nuance to the medical registry–based data as well. Pulling that data together, our best estimate for recurrence rates for *diagnosed* HG is in the range of 15 to 25 percent. In some cases, especially with more mild (but still serious) HG, women may not be diagnosed. The diagnosis, as discussed above, isn't black-and-white. It seems possible (or even likely) that having HG in a first pregnancy increases the risk of serious nausea in a later pregnancy for most women. But it may be that they do not all rise to the level of diagnosis (perhaps due in part to better treatment or awareness).

Overall, the evidence suggests a likely but not certain recurrence risk here. These data on recurrence can also be used to look at prevention. In the Norwegian register study, the authors found a lower risk of recurrence with a new partner (16 percent versus 10 percent).[6] It's unclear why this would be and, for most people, it's not a modifiable risk factor (or not one they would want to modify). The Finnish register study found that smoking during pregnancy lowers the risk.[7] However, smoking during pregnancy is not recommended for a whole host of other reasons, so this is also non-actionable.

Although this is discouraging, within the past few years new findings on HG have opened up possible avenues for both prevention and treatment. In December 2023, a new paper in *Nature* presented a set of evidence on the role of a specific hormone—GDF15—in driving nausea and vomiting in pregnancy.[8] This hormone is created by the fetal-placental unit, and the authors find that when the hormone levels produced are high, nausea is worse. The nausea is especially bad for women whose own naturally occurring levels of this hormone are low. This provides at least a partial explanation for why some women are so much sicker than others.

These new findings are exciting and they suggest directions for research into possible treatments. Exactly what forms these treatments could take are not yet clear, but there is considerable promise where there hasn't been in the past. (Also, interesting side note, the lead author on this research got into studying it because her own HG wasn't taken seriously.)

Treatment

Treatment options for HG do not change in a second or later pregnancy. The biggest change is likely to be that you anticipate the condition and know how to better manage it.

Treating HG is very patient-specific—options include lifestyle changes, medications (like Zofran and others), and in some cases the use of less traditional treatments. Sometimes doctors will consider use of cannabis to treat nausea and vomiting when other medications have failed. Some very small, nonrandomized studies may suggest efficacy.[9] Given other concerns about marijuana use during pregnancy, this approach is not typically recommended and is something that would need to be carefully discussed with your doctor.

Ultimately, if you had HG in a first pregnancy and learned how to partially manage it, that approach may be beneficial again. Being prepared to implement a plan for recurrence is crucial.

MEDICAL PERSPECTIVE

HG is one of the most difficult conditions to treat. It is difficult to predict what treatment might work in one person versus another, and frankly, for the patients with HG, often nothing really "works." A lot of what we are doing with HG is just getting the patient to the next day. Maybe reducing her symptoms a little, maybe making her a little less miserable. Baby steps, baby steps until it starts to get better on its own (hopefully). From time to time, we do find someone who has severe HG and we engage some treatments (which I'll discuss here) and they work really well. So, despite the difficulty, we have hope!

As Emily noted, just from reading the medical literature on this topic, it is hard to estimate the likelihood that HG will recur.

In my own experience, if someone had true HG in their first pregnancy, there is a high chance (greater than 50 percent) that it will recur in the next pregnancy. However, for many or most people who get HG the second time, it is often less severe, mostly because we all know it might be coming, and treatments begin earlier and escalate more aggressively.

For anyone with HG—first time or recurrence—treatments are focused on four components of the problem:

1. Symptoms (nausea, weakness, vomiting)
2. Dehydration
3. Decreased caloric intake
4. Decreased vitamin and mineral intake

While certain treatments may target one of these, in my experience they are all interconnected. For example, if someone is very nauseated and dehydrated, it is pretty clear that if we can help them with their nausea, they will be able to drink and then not be dehydrated. But it is also true that if we treat the dehydration with intravenous fluids, the nausea often improves as well. For this reason, we try to stay on top of all four components, even if one or two seem to be the most severe.

Using this framing, when I see a patient who had HG in a prior pregnancy, the most important step is to make a plan for how we will stay connected and how we will escalate treatment, if necessary.

Typically, if someone has mild nausea and vomiting, we start with simple measures like vitamin B6 and doxylamine. Vitamin B6 is sometimes called pyridoxine. Doxylamine is a sleep medicine also marketed as Unisom. Both can be obtained separately without a prescription or as a combination pill with a prescription. These two together are very effective for mild nausea and vomiting in pregnancy. Interestingly, we don't completely understand why they work in pregnancy or why they don't work for nonpregnant people with nausea.

If you had HG in a first pregnancy, we might still start with this approach in a second pregnancy, since there is a chance symptoms will be controlled with it.

If that is not sufficient, there are many other options, focused on these four key components.

Symptoms are treated aggressively with anti-nausea medications. Patients with HG usually cannot swallow pills, so these need to be given either intravenously (IV), via a subcutaneous pump (under the skin), or by a dissolvable oral tablet or a rectal suppository. Patients often need a form of antacid to reduce pain and irritation in their esophagus and throat from vomiting. Alternative treatments such as acupuncture, hypnosis, or cognitive therapy are not routine, but if they help, great!

Hydration is critical. Fluids by mouth are optimal, if possible, but if someone cannot keep down enough fluid, they would need IV fluids. The people who need IV fluids are often the same ones who need IV medications, so those two recommendations often go together. Logistically, there is some maneuvering that needs to be done to get IV fluids. Someone skilled in putting in an IV needs to place it, and the IV needs

to be replaced every few days to help prevent infection. So people getting IV fluids at home usually also need some form of home-based nursing, or they need to come to a doctor or nurse every few days to get the
IV changed. There are options for longer-term IV lines, but these are
larger, go into bigger veins, and are advanced further into the vein,
which makes them riskier for complications such as infection or blood
clots. It is frequently a tough decision whether it is better to place one of
the long-term IV lines or to use a short-term one and change it every
few days.

For these issues, we can make better decisions when they are discussed in advance. In a crisis moment of severe dehydration, there isn't
necessarily space for good shared decision making around a long-
versus short-term IV. In a prepregnancy visit, it makes sense to talk
through this. Hopefully, it won't be necessary, but if it is, we'll be in a
better position to move quickly in a direction that works for you.

Decreased caloric intake is best helped by getting some form of oral
nutrition, even if it is liquid protein shakes and the like. Amazingly,
people can go a long time with minimal calories if they remain hydrated, so there is wiggle room here. If it comes down to it, sometimes
calories need to be given intravenously (TPN, or total parenteral nutrition), which does require one of the larger, long-term IV lines. Another
option is to place a nasogastric tube (a tube inserted into the nose that
goes all the way down into the stomach or small intestine) and feed
people that way. As you can imagine, it is not pleasant, but many
people do tolerate this, and it tends to be safer and easier than giving
calories intravenously. A greater variety of foods can be fed through a
nasogastric tube, and it does not have the associated risks of infection
and blood clotting of the large IV lines.

Vitamin and mineral intake needs to be monitored. Sometimes a registered clinical dietician or nutritionist is consulted to help calculate what vitamins and minerals need to be supplemented. These can be given orally, often as chewables. If those are not tolerated, they can be given intravenously.

The aforementioned treatments are adjusted frequently until a good regimen is identified, and then monitored for any further adjustments.

As these interventions suggest, treatment of severe HG often requires hospitalization, sometimes for a prolonged period of time. Medication and fluid adjustments are more difficult to do at home, and not everyone has access to home-based nursing care. But ideally the best regimen would allow the patient to be at home.

Usually, we can make things better. For anyone who has any experience with HG, you know that any amount of better is a welcome relief.

Bottom Line

- Diagnosed hyperemesis gravidarum recurs about 25 percent of the time, but some level of recurrence is more common.
- There is little that can be done to prevent HG, but being on top of treatment can improve the experience.
- Ask what monitoring your doctor or midwife will put in place to identify HG early.
- Find out what treatment plan your doctor or midwife will follow if the HG becomes severe.
- Put in place supports to help your family in the event that you are seriously ill.

CHAPTER 5

~~~~~~~~~

First-Trimester Miscarriage

DEFINITION: Loss of a pregnancy within the
first 12 weeks of pregnancy

OVERALL PREVALENCE: Up to 25 percent of pregnancies

RECURRENCE RISK GROUP: Low after one or two;
intermediate after three or more

First-trimester miscarriage is, sadly, extremely common. Studies that detect pregnancies from the moment of conception show loss rates as high as 50 percent, although many of these are losses that occur before you would typically suspect you were pregnant.

A pregnancy can typically be detected by 4, and certainly by 5, gestational weeks (because of the way the counting is done, this is four or five weeks after the start of your last period). For that reason, data can inform us about changes in the risk of pregnancy loss starting at week 5.

The graph on the following page, drawn from a meta-analysis on this topic, shows the remaining risk of miscarriage by week.[1] The horizontal axis shows the week of pregnancy and the vertical axis shows the risk of pregnancy loss moving forward for patients with a viable pregnancy in each week of gestation.

We've ended the graph at 12 weeks. There are four studies covered here; unfortunately, the most reliable one is the one with the largest miscarriage rates. In that study, researchers recruited women in California, targeting them based on early-pregnancy tests in their medical records. Because of this early pregnancy recruitment, they were better able to study risks of loss early on.

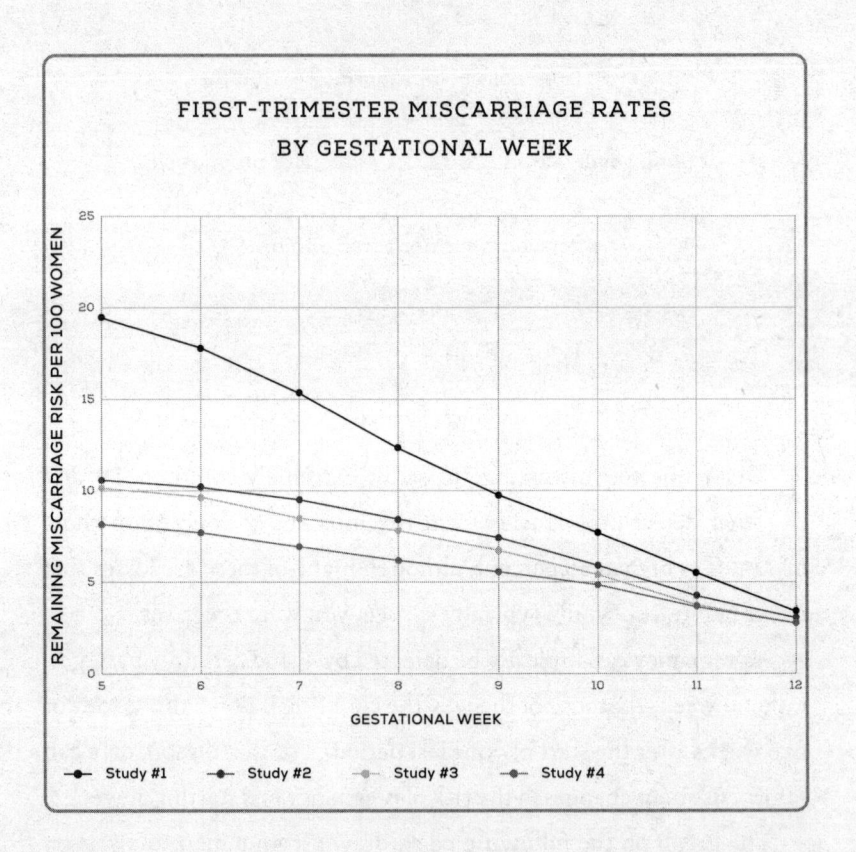

FIRST-TRIMESTER MISCARRIAGE RATES
BY GESTATIONAL WEEK

Focusing on this, most reliable, study, we see clear evidence of a drop in the risk of miscarriage over the first trimester of pregnancy.

Among pregnancies at 5 weeks, perhaps 20 percent will end in miscarriage (it is worth saying: many losses at this point would be to people who didn't even know they were pregnant). By week 9, that figure drops to 10 percent, and by 12 weeks it is less than 5 percent.

The obvious conclusion is that gestational age is one clear determinant of miscarriage risk. Another determinant is maternal age. In a population-based study of over 400,000 pregnancies in Norway, researchers were able to look at miscarriage rates by maternal age.[2] What they observed (graph below) is a risk that is low—about 10 percent in these data—until age thirty-three or so, and then it increases to as high as 50 percent for pregnancies in women over forty-five.

The most important factor in first-trimester pregnancy losses is

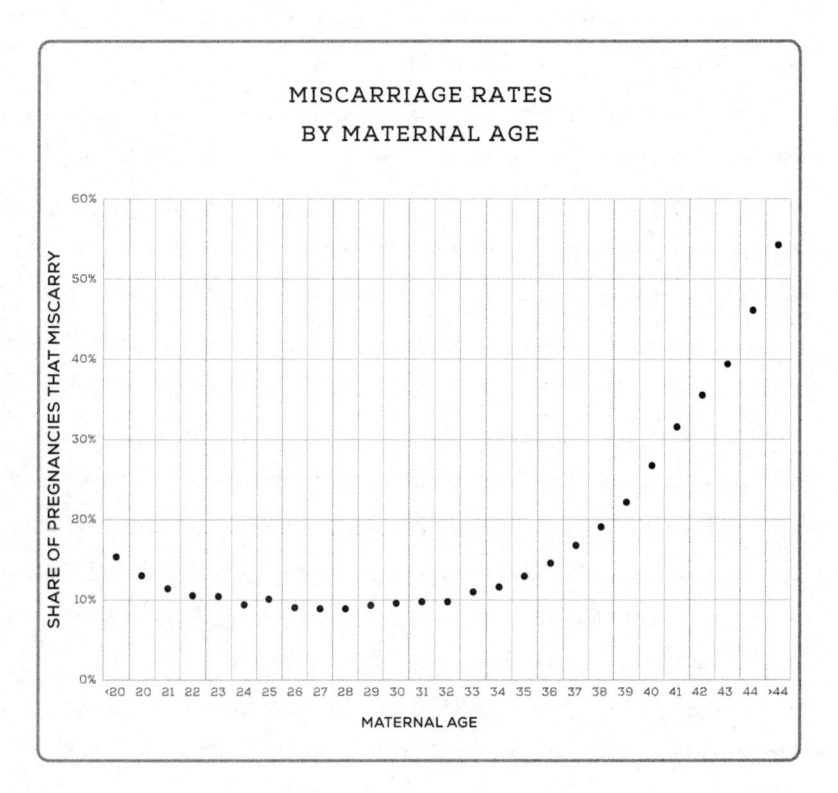

MISCARRIAGE RATES
BY MATERNAL AGE

chromosomal abnormalities. Precise numbers are tricky to find, but it is generally accepted that well over 50 percent and perhaps as much as 90 percent of first-trimester losses are a result of chromosomal abnormalities. This helps us understand both the relationship with gestational age and the relationship with maternal age.

On the first count, since many chromosomal abnormalities are inconsistent with development, they are more likely to miscarry very early in pregnancy. On the second, in general, abnormalities are more likely with older eggs, explaining the role of maternal age.

This information is important in part because it underscores that *for the vast majority of pregnancy losses in the first trimester, there is nothing that you did to cause it or could have done to prevent it.* The miscarriage is unrelated to any behavior or choices you made during pregnancy. It's incredibly sad, but it is not your fault.

A first-trimester miscarriage can be incredibly isolating. The conventional approach to a pregnancy announcement is to tell people only after the first trimester has passed because of the high rate of miscarriage during this trimester. But this means that many people who miscarry find themselves with limited sources of support.

Since I have been writing about pregnancy, I've been heartened to see that discussions about miscarriage have become less taboo. Public figures—from the Duchess of Sussex to comedian Ali Wong—have talked publicly about their pregnancy losses, and their toll. This is a clear first step toward finding support. Better support can only go so far, though. Pregnancy loss comes with the grief and processing that accompanies any loss. And this grief and processing is all the more important if you are contemplating another pregnancy.

In talking with women who lost a pregnancy in the first trimester, I frequently noticed a sense of disconnection with a second pregnancy.

• • •

I had two first-trimester miscarriages before getting pregnant a third time and having my son last year. My partner and I were always paranoid about getting "too excited" during our third pregnancy out of fear something inevitably would go terribly. We waited until 20 weeks to really tell anyone out of fear we'd have to later tell them that, never mind, something bad happened again. I was waiting for something awful to happen more or less my entire pregnancy. We actually agreed the third pregnancy would be our last regardless of the outcome, simply because we couldn't stand the emotional roller coaster anymore. We'd always been interested in adopting anyway, so we figured maybe having our own baby just wasn't meant to be for whatever reason. Even now that we have a healthy baby, we both can't even think about having another because getting pregnant and staying pregnant is so daunting and scary.

• • •

A second common theme was anxiety and fear.

• • •

We had tried for more than six months for baby number two, only to end in miscarriage at 7 weeks. I felt extremely defeated. We tried again after one normal menstrual cycle mainly because it felt like I was starting over and I didn't want to lose more time. It was an extremely emotional time for me. I was lucky enough to get pregnant right away after that (currently 27 weeks), but even then I felt robbed of the joy that comes with early pregnancy. I was so anxious that something would go wrong again.

I didn't tell people; I took pregnancy tests every day for weeks. Even now
I feel somewhat disconnected from this baby because I'm just waiting for
the other shoe to drop.

• • •

Since the cause of a first-trimester miscarriage is rarely confirmed
(genetic abnormalities are usually suspected, but testing is not typically
done after a single miscarriage), there is added anxiety. As one woman
told me: "We tried again mostly because I was able to take solace in
the fact that my OB-GYN thought she knew what had caused my miscarriage and had a plan to possibly keep it from happening a second
time." The identification of a cause is unusual. Without it, fear can
take the place of explanation.

As in many complications, a natural question after a first-trimester
miscarriage as you contemplate trying again might be: *Is it likely to*
happen again? A closely related question is: *What can I do to prevent it?*
For this, we will turn to the data.

WHAT THE DATA SAYS: RECURRENCE AND TREATMENT

Recurrence

As with virtually every pregnancy complication discussed in this book,
having had a miscarriage does raise the risk of miscarriage in a future
pregnancy. Age is one reason for this. Also, a small proportion of mis-

carriages are due to conditions in one or both parents, which would carry from one pregnancy to another.

From the cohort study from Norway discussed earlier, we can also see the risk of repeat miscarriage. Even after controlling for the age of the mother, they estimate that the risk of miscarriage is 1.5 times as high after a single miscarriage, 2.2 times as high after two miscarriages, and 4 times as high after three or more miscarriages. There is a big distinction between the latter two numbers and the former—and after two or more miscarriages, it is clearly appropriate to seek more medical advice.

Having said that, it is worth emphasizing again that miscarriages are so common that the vast majority of people who have one go on to have children. We can see some nice evidence of this in a study that recruited about 53,000 women in Israel at the time they were giving birth and asked them about their prior pregnancies.[3]

Among the women who were giving birth to their first child, 18.5 percent of them had at least one miscarriage before that (and almost 5 percent had more than one). For the women giving birth to their second child, 37 percent had at least one miscarriage. Finally, among women giving birth to their fifth or later child, 70 percent had at least one miscarriage, and one-third had more than one.

A final useful set of data comes from Nate's own practice, published in 2022.[4] In this study, Nate and his coauthors looked at how miscarriage rates varied by gestational age and number of prior miscarriages, *but only in women with an ultrasound verifying a viable pregnancy.* That is, they asked about the risks of miscarriage among women at, say, 8 weeks of pregnancy, if they had an ultrasound verifying that a pregnancy was developing normally at that week.

The table on the following page shows these findings. There are higher miscarriage rates for people with prior miscarriages, but they also decline a lot as the pregnancy progresses.

Predicted Risk of Miscarriage In Viable Pregnancies, Based on Gestational Age and Number of Prior Miscarriages

Gestational Age	Number of Prior Miscarriages			
	0	1	2	3+
6 weeks	8.3%	13.3%	21.1%	33.7%
7 weeks	6.0%	9.6%	15.2%	24.3%
8 weeks	4.3%	6.9%	11.0%	17.5%
9 weeks	3.1%	5.0%	7.9%	12.6%
10 weeks	2.2%	3.6%	5.7%	9.1%
11 weeks	1.6%	2.6%	4.1%	6.6%
12 weeks	1.2%	1.9%	3.0%	4.7%
13 weeks	0.8%	1.3%	2.1%	3.4%

The natural next question, then, is when to try again. Unfortunately, there is no clear guidance. People are often told to wait, but there is actually no specific medical reason for that. Having a normal period before trying again would make a subsequent pregnancy easier to date, but that is a fairly minor consideration. The American College of Obstetricians and Gynecologists simply says that there is no evidence-based advice, while also noting that it may be a good idea to abstain from sex for a few weeks in order to avoid infection risks.[5]

The most important consideration here is whether you feel ready. In some cases, this is right away. In others, it is not. If you're not ready, wait. If you are, then go ahead and try.

Treatment

As noted, most miscarriages in the first trimester are due to genetic abnormalities. Since these often occur at random, after a single miscarriage usually no additional testing or treatments will be recommended. It's true that the risk of a second miscarriage is slightly elevated, but this elevation is small, and given the large share of women who will go on to have a healthy second pregnancy, usually it makes sense to try again before delving into further testing.

After multiple miscarriages, additional testing is likely necessary. You may find that you have one of the rare complications that increases recurrent miscarriage risk.

One of these conditions is a uterine abnormality called a uterine septum, in which the top portion of the uterine cavity is divided into two spaces by an extra band of tissue. This is estimated to occur in 5 to 10 percent of women with recurrent miscarriage.[6] A second condition is antiphospholipid antibody syndrome (APS), which is a relatively rare autoimmune disorder (1 in 2,000 people), but is most common in women of reproductive age. It can lead to blood clots, as well as numerous complications of pregnancy such as miscarriage, preeclampsia, fetal growth restriction, and stillbirth. It is usually treated with low-dose aspirin and injectable anticoagulants, such as heparin.

Some people may also have an increased risk of chromosomal abnormalities. One reason for this—already discussed—is age. A second possibility is a condition called balanced translocation, which affects about 1 in 400 people.[7] This is a genetic phenomenon in which a person has the correct total number of chromosomes, but a portion of two of them have changed places. For example, a small piece of DNA from your 22nd chromosome is swapped with a piece on the 13th. For you, this is not a problem: you have all the genes you need, they are just not on quite the right chromosome.

However, this presents an issue for fertility. Each parent passes along one copy of each chromosome. If you pass the copy of the 22nd that is missing the DNA but you *do not* pass the copy of the 13th that has that missing piece, the fetus will end up totally missing that gene. This can cause pregnancy loss.

A balanced translocation can be detected through genetic testing of parents. For either of these issues, the treatment approach would be IVF with preimplantation genetic testing (PGT). This approach, while time-consuming, expensive, and taxing, can select embryos that are viable.

MEDICAL PERSPECTIVE

I have heard from countless patients that having a miscarriage, in addition to it being very sad and painful, can also be very frustrating. There are a lot of mixed messages from doctors, and it can sometimes feel like nobody has any answers. This is in part because, despite how common miscarriage is, there is a lot we do not understand about early pregnancy and miscarriage.

When I see someone with one or more prior pregnancy losses, the main question I try to answer is: What is the likelihood that this loss is due to a genetic abnormality in the embryo? If it is likely, there is no reason to do additional tests and certainly no reason to recommend any treatments or procedures (the one exception would be from a balanced translocation).

This crucial question is not always easy to answer. I will typically start by thinking through the following questions:

1. *At what gestational age was the pregnancy loss?* The earlier the loss, the more likely it was due to a genetic abnormality. In this discussion, it is important to clarify how certain you are about the timing of a loss. For example, if someone has an ultrasound at 12 weeks showing a nonviable embryo measuring 7 weeks with no heartbeat, I would consider this a 7-week loss, not a 12-week loss. Earlier ultrasounds for dating can be helpful in establishing this, if available.

2. *Was genetic testing done on the pregnancy loss?* If someone has a pregnancy loss, the tissue can sometimes be sent for genetic testing to assess whether there is a normal chromosomal makeup. This is straightforward to do if someone chooses a surgical approach to miscarriage (a dilation and curettage). If a miscarriage is managed at home, saving tissue for genetic testing can be incredibly difficult emotionally. It may be valuable, though, especially after multiple losses.

3. *How many losses have you had?* As noted, the vast majority of single losses are due to a random genetic abnormality that is not likely to repeat. With each additional loss, the chance that there is another cause (either a systematic genetic issue or something else) goes up. In these cases, we typically do more testing.

This distinction is often not explained well by doctors. Sometimes the messaging received is: *You don't need a workup because you had only one miscarriage. If you lose one or two more, we will run some tests.* Yes, this does sound like you don't deserve testing until you've had several losses. In truth, if I run a bunch of tests on everyone with one loss, a fair percentage will get abnormal tests. For most of these people, the abnormal test is a coincidence, not a cause. We are therefore cautious in running a huge panel of tests on a patient unless we are reasonably confident that an abnormal test has a high probability of being the cause of the loss and warrants treatment.

Answering these three questions, as well as performing an overall assessment of someone's medical, surgical, and pregnancy history, will often help me decide if someone needs additional testing or treatments, and which ones.

For women with three losses, or other circumstances suggestive of a cause other than bad luck, some of the tests I might recommend are:

- Chromosomal analysis of both parents (blood test) to test for a balanced translocation in either parent
- Testing for antiphospholipid antibody syndrome (blood test)
- Assessment of the uterine cavity, which can be done in the following ways:
  - Saline infusion sonohysterogram, or SIS (a specialized ultrasound done after inserting some sterile water into the uterus through the cervix)
  - MRI
  - Hysterosalpingogram, or HSG (an X-ray of the uterus after injecting a dye into the uterus through the cervix. This is the test also used to assess the fallopian tubes in an infertility workup)

If one of these tests reveals an abnormality, treatment options will depend on what was found. For a balanced translocation, often the treatment is IVF and preimplantation genetic testing of the embryos. For antiphospholipid antibody syndrome, the treatment is low-dose aspirin and sometimes injectable blood thinners. For a uterine septum, surgical removal via hysteroscopy (a camera through the cervix) might be recommended.

Most of the time, all the tests will be normal (this is true in my experience, but also statistically expected given that these known causes are rare). That is great news, but it can also be disconcerting, as we are left with a situation where we think there may be something other than bad luck going on but we can't figure out what it is. In general, most data shows that even with three or more losses, with a normal workup the chances of a future successful pregnancy are very good, and if people "keep trying," it should eventually work out.

That said, people in this situation are understandably frustrated and sometimes desperate to find "something," and continue to go from doctor to doctor until one finds something wrong and recommends a treatment. There are many treatments, including ones targeted at the immune system (immunoglobulin, intralipids, steroids, immune modulators), as well as blood thinners (with the exception being treatment for antiphospholipid antibody syndrome) that are prescribed in this space but that don't have statistical backing. On the one hand, maybe that doctor will find something rare and pursue an unproven treatment, and their treatment will work for you. On the other hand, you may be given a diagnosis that has nothing to do with the losses and a recommendation to start treatments that are complex, potentially harmful, expensive, and not going to improve your chances of success. So the stakes are high. Unfortunately, we just don't have enough data to be conclusive in many cases.

But there are three things that we do know: (1) the majority of mis-carriages are due to a genetic abnormality in the embryo (it's not your fault); (2) practically without exception, miscarriage is *not* due to something the mother did or did not do (it's not your fault); and (3) with time, continued trying, and sometimes interventions, nearly all people will have a successful pregnancy (there is every reason to be optimistic). So feel sad, even angry. But don't feel guilty. Also, try not to lose hope. We're here to help.

Bottom Line

- There is a mildly elevated risk of miscarriage after one loss; this is more elevated after two or three losses.
- Nearly all losses in the first trimester—including repeated losses—are a result of genetic abnormalities.
- Most people with one or two losses don't need a workup, as an abnormal result is more likely to be a coincidence and not the cause of the miscarriage(s).
- There are a few known causes of recurrent losses that are potentially amenable to treatment.
- Be cautious of unproven treatments.

Second- and Third-Trimester Complications

CHAPTER 6

Second-Trimester Miscarriage

DEFINITION: Loss of a pregnancy between 12 and 20 weeks of pregnancy

OVERALL PREVALENCE: 1 to 2 percent

RECURRENCE RISK GROUP: Low (typically less than 5 percent)

There are at least three important differences between first- and second-trimester miscarriages.

First, second-trimester miscarriages are much less common—while perhaps a quarter of conceptions are lost in the first trimester, second-trimester miscarriage rates are in the range of 1 to 2 percent.

A 2012 meta-analysis on this topic combined four studies that estimate miscarriage rates over the course of pregnancy.[1] In a prior chapter, we showed the graph up to 12 weeks; on the next page is the graph after 12 weeks. The risk continues to go down over the second trimester, but the scale of the graph here is much smaller than in the first trimester.

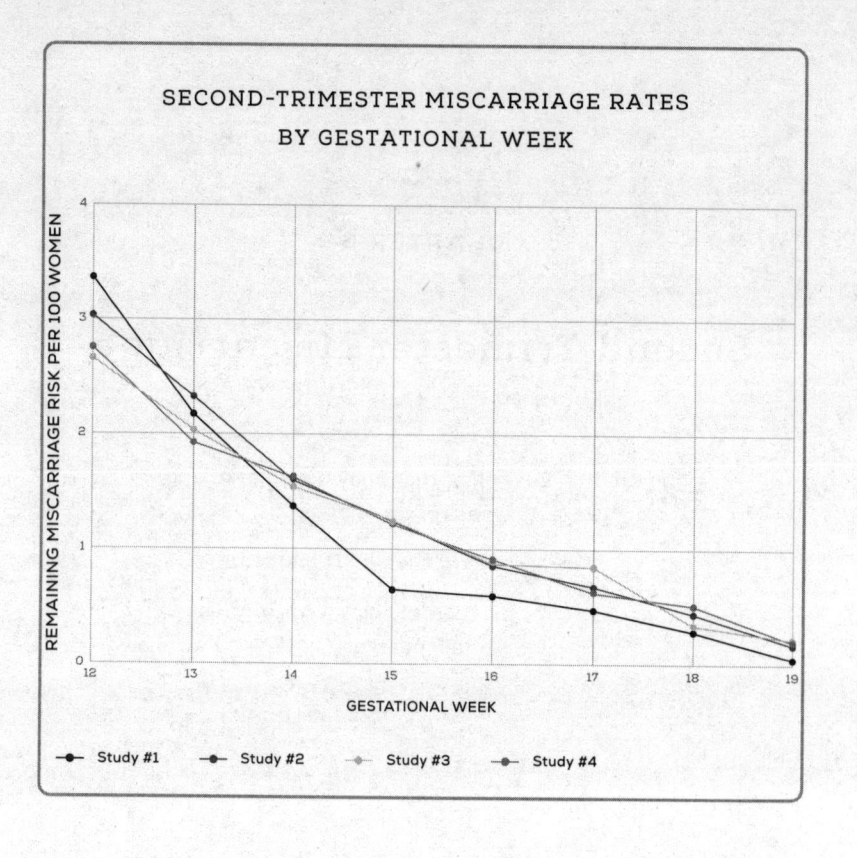

Next, second-trimester miscarriages are often much, much harder than first-trimester miscarriages. By the second trimester, most people have announced a pregnancy and may be starting to show. A loss at this point is often more public. In some cases, this can elicit more support, but those feelings are not uncomplicated. As one woman told me:

• • •

I've always told people pretty quickly in the past about my pregnancies. While I don't regret this, it was nice to have the support, it was REALLY

hard to know everyone was thinking about my loss. I don't do well in a
crisis feeling like a victim.

• • •

Physically, the recovery from a pregnancy loss in this time period is also more complex.

Finally—and here is the better news—second-trimester miscarriages are less likely to be caused by genetic anomalies and more likely to be the result of a condition that can be identified and treated. This means a lower recurrence risk and more that can be done. That's what we'll focus on in this chapter.

Before getting into causes, we should define what we mean by second-trimester miscarriage. Technically, any birth or loss prior to 20 weeks is a miscarriage, and any birth or loss at 20 weeks or more is considered a preterm birth or stillbirth. However, the second trimester extends until 24 or 26 weeks. Part of the reason for this discrepancy is that some babies born between 20 and 24 weeks survive (about 0 percent at 20 weeks and up to 50 percent or more at 24 weeks), so it would be wrong to characterize a birth that resulted in a live baby that survived as a "miscarriage." So we are considering a second-trimester miscarriage as a loss between 12 and 20 weeks.

In some cases, a miscarriage may not be detected until 12 or 13 weeks of pregnancy, but the fetus's measurements indicate that it stopped developing earlier. In these cases, it would be defined as a first-trimester miscarriage, even if the detection is later.

Between 12 and 20 weeks, there can be two types of miscarriages. One type is a fetal demise that could be discovered by ultrasound, or can trigger preterm labor and delivery of a nonviable baby. The second type is when the primary issue is (very) premature labor and the baby dies either during labor or after birth. It is usually possible to differentiate between these two types, but sometimes it is not. For example, if someone presents at 18 weeks in labor with an 18-week-sized fetus that is not alive, it usually would not be known which happened first—the labor or the demise.

A second-trimester miscarriage is usually more complicated medically than a first-trimester loss. With a first-trimester miscarriage, most patients are given the option to wait for the fetus to pass on its own, take medication to expedite the passing, or undergo a dilation and curettage (D&C) procedure, sometimes also called a dilation and aspiration (D&A). This involves dilating the cervix enough to pass a small tube into the uterus to remove the nonviable pregnancy. These are all generally safe procedures in the first trimester, and most OB-GYNs are trained to do a D&C at this stage if that is what you choose.

In the second trimester, there are fewer options. It is rarely wise to wait for a fetus to pass on its own or to take medications to have it pass at home. The larger size of the fetus and the placenta raise concerns about pain, excess bleeding, and retained placental material.

A second-trimester miscarriage requires either an induction of labor (and delivery) in the hospital, or a more advanced surgical procedure to remove the fetus and placenta. The second-trimester correlation to a D&C is a procedure called a dilation and extraction or dilation and evacuation (D&E). Both a D&C and a D&E involve dilating the cervix, but in the second trimester, since a larger fetus has to be removed, the cervix needs to be dilated more and larger instruments need to be used. This surgical procedure therefore is more risky, takes a lot of training and skill to perform safely, sometimes takes a few days of preparation (to soften and open the cervix), and most OB-GYNs are not trained to do this.

Making this often more challenging is that as a patient, you'll often be asked what approach you want to take (labor and delivery versus a D&E). There is no easy way to choose. One woman, reflecting later, told me:

• • •

My only other thought, now being a mother, is that I might prefer to birth the baby rather than have a D&E if something like this happened again. I wasn't given the option to hold her after the procedure. I mourn the fact I never got to look at the daughter I lost. At the time, I wanted to pretend it never happened.

• • •

All there is to say is to give yourself grace—there are no easy choices.

Also, after a second-trimester loss, whether induced or removed through the surgical procedure, the physical recovery is somewhere between a first-trimester loss and a full-term birth. Many women produce breast milk after a second-trimester loss, which causes both physical discomfort and frequently a lot of emotional pain as well.

Moving from a second-trimester loss to trying for a later pregnancy adds physical recovery to the already difficult emotional recovery. You may be physically ready to consider another pregnancy far before you are emotionally ready. And the challenges in a second pregnancy may be difficult to predict; when I talked to women about this, unexpected challenges emerged as a common theme.

. . .

We were set on trying again. While trying to conceive, I was more relaxed than with prior pregnancies—less ovulation testing and more wait-and-see. The mental overhead of worrying about getting and staying pregnant was too much, so I had to put it in a box in my mind and set it aside. Then I became pregnant and did a complete 180; I used a fetal Doppler every day once I could find the heartbeat, I scheduled appointments as close together as I could, and I was consumed with worry. It was a very lonely and isolating time.

When I returned to work, it was remarkable how being in that space (where I hadn't been since being pregnant) brought my anxious pre-birth feelings rushing back. Like, when I was pregnant I kept telling myself and others I was doing well and felt good and all the positive things. But boy was I a ball of anxiety on the inside—waaaay more so than I even realized. Just a constant underlying tinge of anxiety—what I often hear is the norm for the first pregnancy after a loss.

. . .

For many, a second-trimester miscarriage will bring on additional doctor visits in later pregnancies, and possibly a new set of doctors. As one woman told me:

. . .

I had so much fear and anxiety around the second pregnancy after our late loss in the first. It just felt like the scariest thing to try again. As a result, I was much more empowered the second time to demand additional doctor appointments to ensure I felt like I knew what was happening and had some semblance of control.

• • •

Control may be easier to deliver after a second-trimester loss because the causes are more likely to be identifiable. And, in most cases, they are either unlikely to recur or there is some potentially effective treatment.

WHAT THE DATA SAYS: RECURRENCE AND TREATMENT

In the case of second-trimester miscarriage, recurrence and treatment is largely specific to the possible causes. In the medical perspective in this chapter, Nate will talk through these possible causes in detail, and what treatments may be appropriate.

As an overall summary: many of the causes of second-trimester miscarriage (infection, issues with the placenta) are usually sporadic and not related to any underlying condition. It's therefore unlikely they would occur again—not much more likely than if this had not happened. In these cases, there is no additional medical treatment necessary, although counseling and more prenatal visits for reassurance may be very important and of huge value.

Second-trimester miscarriage can be a result of cervical insufficiency, which would be likely to recur. This has a clear treatment: putting a stitch in the cervix, called a cerclage, which is an effective treatment for this condition.

Finally, second-trimester miscarriage can reflect (very) preterm labor; in this case, treatments like progesterone may be considered.

Overall, in most cases, a second-trimester loss is very unlikely to recur and, in the cases where the cause is known and may recur, we have some treatments. This is positive news.

MEDICAL PERSPECTIVE

Patients I see with a prior second-trimester loss are often in a fog afterward, trying to sort out what happened. They may not have been told, for instance, whether the baby died and then delivered, or if the baby delivered and then died. That uncertainty compounds the difficulties of the way forward. So, much of the conversation I have with patients about a second-trimester loss usually focuses on trying to identify a cause, or at least a few potential ones from a relatively long list of possible causes, which are similar to those that lead to preterm birth or stillbirth.

In brief, there are a few causes that are most common.

Cervical Insufficiency

This topic is covered at length in chapter 10, Preterm Birth. In short, if the cervix dilates earlier than full term, this can cause preterm birth. If it happens very long before term, it can result in a second-trimester miscarriage. For a second-trimester loss, cervical insufficiency would be suspected if there was evidence of painless cervical shortening and dilation after 16 weeks prior to any bleeding, contractions, fetal demise, and delivery. It is rarely the cause of a loss prior to 16 weeks, but it is possible.

Preterm Labor/Premature Rupture of the Membranes

Technically, preterm labor occurs only after 20 weeks, but there are likely a few women who have the same process and deliver at 18 or 19 weeks.

Infection

An infection, either recognized or not, could lead to a second-trimester miscarriage. This could be seen either as a fetal demise or as an early birth. Typically, this is suspected as a cause only if someone has clear signs of infection—fever, pain, or bad-smelling amniotic fluid. This cause is rare.

Placental Insufficiency

This is a cause of second-trimester miscarriage usually presenting as a fetal demise. Prior to the demise, there is usually evidence of placental insufficiency, including a smaller-than-expected fetus, low amniotic fluid, and potentially other sonographic features (echogenic or bright fetal bowel, for example, or abnormal umbilical-cord blood flow). While this is usually sporadic, one potential cause of it that can recur is antiphospholipid antibody syndrome. Antiphospholipid antibody syndrome is a relatively rare autoimmune disorder (1 in 2,000 people), but is most common in women of reproductive age. It can lead to blood clots as well as numerous complications of pregnancy such as miscarriage, preeclampsia, fetal growth restriction, and stillbirth. It is usually treated with low-dose aspirin and injectable anticoagulants, such as heparin.

Testing for this involves bloodwork done at least twice, several months apart, and the tests need to be consistently abnormal to make the diagnosis.

Placental Abruption, Bleeding

This can cause a second-trimester loss through fetal demise or preterm labor. It is nearly always preceded by on-and-off bleeding, sometimes for many weeks. On ultrasound, there may or may not be a collection of blood seen at the edge of the placenta, called a subchorionic hematoma.

A placental abruption can also be caused by trauma—a car accident, for example—and the cause would be clear in this case.

Genetic or Anatomic Fetal Anomaly

A genetic or anatomic anomaly in the fetus can cause a fetal demise and can also lead to premature labor (through an uncertain mechanism). Sometimes these are identified in advance from genetic screening, genetic testing, or ultrasound. But often it is not identified until after the loss by testing of the placenta or fetus, including autopsy.

Genetic causes for miscarriage are less common in the second trimester than the first, but they can still occur. As is the case in the first trimester, these genetic anomalies often occur at random.

Umbilical Cord Complications

Sometimes the umbilical cord can be compressed for a prolonged period of time, leading to a fetal demise in the second trimester. This is typically unpredictable and unpreventable, and often not known to be the cause until other causes have been ruled out.

. . .

With these possible causes in mind, the way I start this conversation with patients is simply asking them to tell their full story. Once I've listened, I ask a lot of follow-up questions to make sure I have the full picture. Important ones include: At what gestational age did it happen? Was the first event a fetal demise or labor? Was there bleeding or cervical changes prior? Was there a genetic or anatomic abnormality or an infection? I ask the patient and anyone else who was with her at the time and might remember certain details. I try to review all the medical records, including doctor notes, laboratory results, ultrasound reports, genetic screening and testing, and, if there was a pathologic examination of the placenta and fetus, those reports as well. If I have never met the patient before, it sometimes takes a few meetings before all this information is collected, so it is ideal if you can try to gather all of it prior to planning for the next pregnancy.

For the same reason, if someone is unfortunately in the middle of a second-trimester loss, it is important to try to understand in real time what is happening and to try to clarify it with the doctor who is treating you. I strongly recommend genetic testing of the fetus or the placenta, as well as pathologic examination of the placenta and fetus. The likelihood of finding a cause is greatly increased (though not assured) if a thorough workup is done at the time. Autopsy is understandably a difficult decision for parents. I do recommend autopsy to increase the chances of finding a cause, but I also totally understand that for some people this will simply not feel possible.

If I see a patient with a past second-trimester loss who is *not* yet pregnant again, I will sometimes recommend a saline infusion sonohysterogram (SIS) or an MRI to assess the shape of the uterine cavity for any possible uterine anomalies. Unless you had clear cervical insufficiency, I will usually recommend testing for antiphospholipid antibody syndrome, and potentially other thrombophilia testing. I will also recommend expanded genetic carrier screening for you and possibly your partner. Exactly what I recommend depends on the details of what happened.

For example, if the second-trimester loss was due to something related to preterm labor, premature rupture of the membranes, or cervical insufficiency, I would want to assess the shape of the uterus in between pregnancies to make sure that isn't a potential cause of the loss. In the second pregnancy, I am going to focus on screening for infection, the role of progesterone, and serial screening of the cervical length (more on these in chapter 10, Preterm Birth). But, if the second-trimester loss was due to a placental problem, like placental insufficiency or abruption, I am going to test for antiphospholipid antibody syndrome between pregnancies and then during the next pregnancy focus on placental function by measuring fetal growth and amniotic fluid volume.

We usually recommend low-dose aspirin and serial ultrasound evaluation, either to check the cervical length, to follow fetal growth, or simply to provide reassurance.

Certainly, for anyone with a prior second-trimester loss, much of the focus in the next pregnancy is on mental health, specifically anxiety and fear over it happening again. This is addressed in more detail in chapter 13, Stillbirth, and the same principles apply.

Taken together, the pregnancy following a second-trimester loss is most often a difficult pregnancy emotionally, but the prognosis is typically very optimistic, and the pregnancy most often ends with an uncomplicated, healthy birth.

Bottom Line

- Second-trimester miscarriages are more likely than first to have a known cause.
- Treating this cause can dramatically lower the risk of recurrence.
- Finding out the details of what happened is particularly important but can sometimes be very challenging.
- Whether the loss was due to a fetal demise, preterm labor, or cervical insufficiency is key.
- Your doctor or midwife will tailor testing and treatment to the specific cause of the second-trimester loss.

~~~~~~~~~

CHAPTER 7

Gestational Diabetes

DEFINITION: Diabetes diagnosed during pregnancy,
without a diagnosis before

OVERALL PREVALENCE: About 8 percent of
pregnancies in the US

RECURRENCE RISK GROUP: High (more than 50 percent)

O ur focus in this chapter is on gestational diabetes—diabetes that is diagnosed during pregnancy. Before getting into this, it is worth noting that you can also have diabetes before pregnancy. If this is the case, it's very important to find treatment that gets your diabetes under control (with a lower A1C measure) before getting pregnant again. In particular, when this measure is elevated above 7 percent, the risk of birth defects is significantly higher.

If you do not have known diabetes before pregnancy, you'll be tested during pregnancy—typically at the beginning of the third trimester (24 to 28 weeks). The test for gestational diabetes will be familiar to nearly everyone who has been pregnant. Diagnosis of this condition in the US, at least, is done through universal screening with a glucose challenge. One morning, midpregnancy, you fast and then drink a terrible glucose drink. (Nate tells me you do not necessarily have to fast for this test! I feel cheated.) My drink was orange and I still remember gagging it down in the car on the way to the doctor. She told me it would "be better cold"; I guess it's hard to judge without the comparison.

An hour after consuming the glucose drink, your blood sugar is tested. If the glucose is above a certain level, you are either diagnosed directly with gestational diabetes or (more commonly) tested again using a three-hour waiting period (with four blood draws—yes, four).

There are two reasons that universal screening is recommended for this condition. One is that gestational diabetes is quite common. In 2020, an estimated 7.8 percent of births were complicated by gestational diabetes.[1] With these high rates, it makes sense to test the whole population. The second reason is that, when appropriately recognized, gestational diabetes can be well managed during pregnancy and usually does not lead to serious adverse effects for you or the baby. This dramatically increases the value of diagnosing it.

Gestational diabetes is diagnosed in any pregnant woman who has glucose levels above the cutoff after the screening tests. But from the standpoint of understanding recurrence and health risks, it is very important to distinguish two groups.

First, there is a group of women who enter pregnancy with diabetes, or borderline diabetes, which they were not aware of, and who are diagnosed during pregnancy. Pregnancy is often a time of increased interaction with the medical system, so it is not surprising that non-pregnancy medical issues that may have gone undiagnosed before may be recognized during this period.

Second, there is a group of women who entered pregnancy with normal blood sugar, but the hormones of the placenta affect their processing of blood sugar, making their blood glucose higher. In fact, nearly *all* pregnant women have some increase in glucose from the placenta, but we call it gestational diabetes when it crosses a certain threshold. In an ideal world, there would be language to distinguish this group from the first group, but for historical reasons these are defined together.

This distinction is important for two reasons. The first is that these groups have different risks for complications. Anyone with high blood sugar in pregnancy, for any reason, has an increased risk of having a baby who is large for gestational age. This can increase the risk of cesarean delivery and shoulder dystocia (when the baby's shoulder gets caught above the mother's pubic bone in childbirth). High blood sugar also increases the risk of neonatal hypoglycemia (low blood sugar) after birth.

However, for individuals in the first group who have undiagnosed prepregnancy diabetes, there are also higher risks of preeclampsia and stillbirth.[2]

The second reason this is an important distinction is that it has a large impact on recurrence risk. If you were tested after pregnancy and confirmed not to have any baseline glucose intolerance or diabetes, the recurrence risk of gestational diabetes is lower, whereas if you have actual diabetes or borderline diabetes, the recurrence risk is much higher.

The problem is that when we diagnose someone with gestational diabetes, we often don't know which group they are in at the time. After pregnancy, it is possible to retest for diabetes, which will help us better understand if the pregnancy was the cause of the high blood sugar. During pregnancy, there are some clues, but we cannot be sure. So, for anyone diagnosed with diabetes in pregnancy it is called, by definition, gestational diabetes. We know that some patients likely have some form of glucose intolerance, or borderline diabetes, or actual diabetes, but we can't really sort it out until after delivery. So, we treat everyone with gestational diabetes like they have diabetes and increase the intensity of this based on the level of the blood sugars.

With this background, we can turn to the data, which will give us some sense of the numbers for overall estimated recurrence risk and for treatment.

WHAT THE DATA SAYS: RECURRENCE AND TREATMENT

Recurrence

The risk of recurrence for gestational diabetes in a later pregnancy is high. A 2007 review put it between 30 and 84 percent.[3] This full range is a bit misleading. The one study with the very high rate—84 percent—had only nineteen patients and the confidence interval is extremely wide.

Putting that one study aside, the remaining studies show recurrence in a lower range, but with significant variation by racial group. For studies limited to non-Hispanic white women, the range is 30 to 40 percent recurrence. For studies that were predominantly women of color (Black, Hispanic, Asian), the recurrence range is 50 to 70 percent.

These figures are in line with a more recent review (from 2015), which showed a pooled recurrence risk of 48 percent, with lower risks for non-Hispanic white women.[4]

Beyond recurrence, many people are interested in whether severity of the condition in a first pregnancy predicts severity or recurrence in a second. With gestational diabetes, the obvious way to measure severity is with the glucose test counts, but unfortunately, those results are not included in the data. However, we can see the use of insulin in the data, and from that we can conclude that individuals who use insulin in a first pregnancy (which is associated with more serious disease) have higher rates of recurrence.[5]

So it seems likely that greater severity would be associated with both a greater risk of recurrence and a greater risk of more severe recurrence, but we cannot see that directly in the data at present.

An important point, related to this discussion: if you retest for diabetes after pregnancy and still have it, it is likely that you had diabetes before pregnancy and that it wasn't a result of your pregnancy. In that case, your risk of recurrence is extremely high—effectively 100 percent—since you actually had diabetes going into the first pregnancy and that remains true going into the next.

A related point about recurrence is that anyone with a history of gestational diabetes has an increased risk of developing overt diabetes in their lifetime, even later in life. It is not exactly clear why this is. It may simply reflect that risk factors for gestational diabetes and diabetes overlap, but one hypothesis is that pregnancy acts as a "window" into your future health. Regardless of the reason, if you have a history of gestational diabetes, it is something you should share early on with all your medical providers, not just obstetricians.

Treatment

The primary interventions for preventing gestational diabetes are similar to those for dealing with type 2 diabetes: diet and exercise. There are a number of randomized trials evaluating diet and exercise interventions during pregnancy. A review paper (a paper that combines results from many other papers) including trials with over 15,000 women found that both diet and exercise interventions (independently or mixed) reduced the incidence of gestational diabetes, by about 24 percent.[6]

Notable in these data are that interventions with exercise alone have the largest estimated effects. Generally, these interventions include moderate-intensity exercise, two or three times a week, for an hour. This is useful to emphasize because often "diet and exercise" are put together as a package, and the reality is that changing one's diet (during pregnancy or at any time) is difficult. Many people may find it more feasible to exercise than to significantly diet during pregnancy.

If you had gestational diabetes in a prior pregnancy and you do not currently exercise, beginning moderate aerobic activity is an evidence-based preventive step you can take now.

If you are going to work to change your diet, a choice with some support in the data is the Mediterranean diet. A 2022 study that compared outcomes across women found that those with a greater adherence to this diet had lower rates of gestational diabetes (about 35 percent less).[7]

The obvious concern in a study like this is that the group who adheres more closely to the diet is different in other ways. That's true in the data, but in this study as you add more controls for differences across groups, the association actually gets *stronger*. This makes the claim for a causal relationship more compelling. You can see this in the graph below—when adjusted for control variables, the differences are both larger and more consistent.

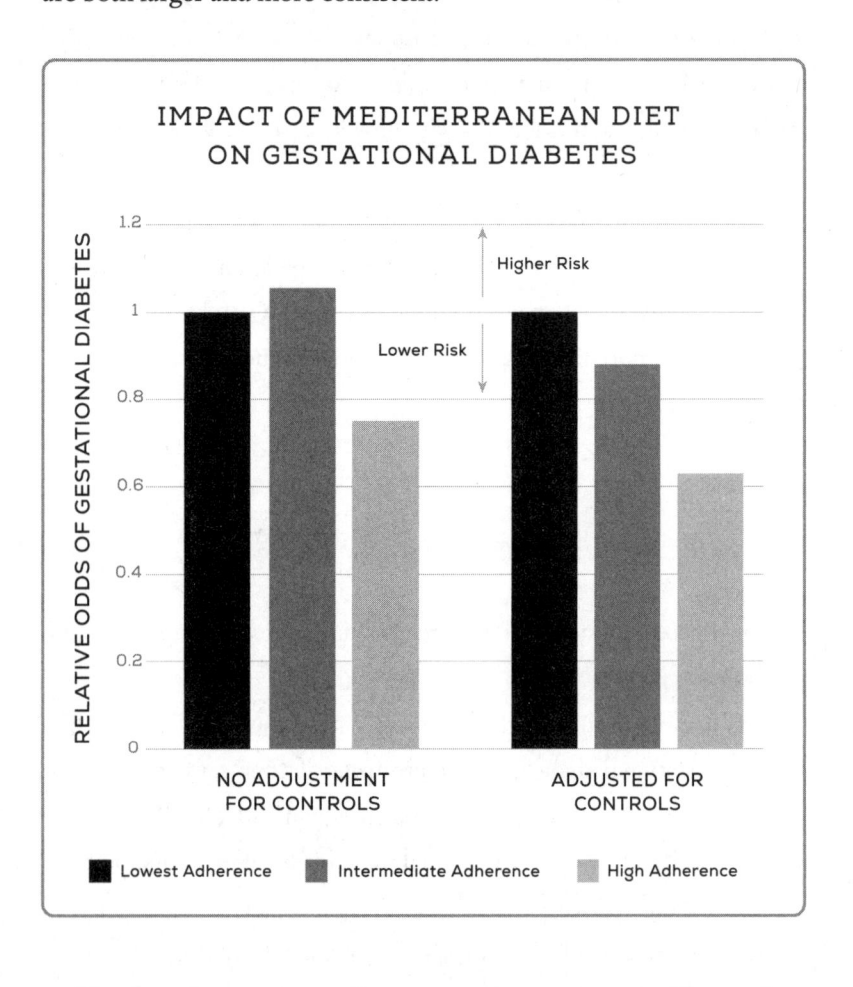

IMPACT OF MEDITERRANEAN DIET
ON GESTATIONAL DIABETES

The data does not strongly support other treatments. The medication metformin has been used to prevent or treat diabetes outside pregnancy, but the one randomized controlled trial in pregnancy did not find significant impacts.[8] This trial did not include very many people, which made it difficult to detect small effects. There may be more exploration of that treatment over time.

In the similarly speculative camp, there is some recent evidence that supplementation with myo-inositol, a type of vitamin B, could lead to dramatic decreases in gestational diabetes (in a meta-analysis of four trials, this is estimated to be up to 70 percent).[9] However, these trials are small, and this is still a very new idea, so we do not have conclusive evidence.

As with other conditions, a final important intervention is simply better monitoring. The most significant complications of gestational diabetes come only when it is poorly controlled. If you know your risk is higher, it is more likely that the condition will be detected and controlled earlier.

MEDICAL PERSPECTIVE

For most people, gestational diabetes is a nuisance condition, but not a dangerous one.

The most important part of my visit with someone who has a history of gestational diabetes is determining if they have diabetes or borderline diabetes when they are not pregnant. Ideally, I would see someone with a history of gestational diabetes *between* pregnancies so we can test during that period.

Most of my patients are surprised to hear me say this. They have heard forever that "diabetes is really bad" and they assume that since they now have diabetes it's going to be dangerous to them and the baby. So, I usually spend the first part of the consultation explaining a lot of the background detailed in this chapter. For most women, gestational diabetes is a slight over-response to the placental hormones, leading to slightly higher than normal glucose levels in pregnancy that *might* have an impact on the baby, and so for that reason we try to get those glucose levels back to normal, or mostly normal. That's about it. It would be great if we could rename gestational diabetes something like "hyperglycemia of pregnancy" or "sorry-you-need-to-prick-your-finger-four-times-a-day-syndrome."

For about 80 percent of women with gestational diabetes, all they need to do is modify their diet to achieve normal, or mostly normal, blood glucose. This includes eating fewer carbohydrates and more protein and fat, and trying to substitute complex carbs for simple carbs (like whole wheat bread instead of white bread). For the 20 percent of women for whom this is not enough, we usually recommend medication to help lower the blood sugar. This is usually done with injections of insulin but sometimes can be achieved with pills taken once or twice a day.

It's not that we don't take gestational diabetes seriously, but we try to be precise about the actual severity of the problem, the potential consequences, and the necessary steps to take. The same is true when trying to determine if it is going to happen again in the next pregnancy, and how much that matters.

There are two ways to test for diabetes outside pregnancy. One is a test for hemoglobin A1C, which is a good marker for glucose levels over the recent few months or so. The A1C test measures what percentage of your hemoglobin is *glycosylated* (has a sugar attached to it). The more sugar in your blood and the longer it persists, the higher this percentage is. So, it is a good assessment of your sugar levels over a longish period of time. It's a standard test for diabetes outside pregnancy, and the results can be divided into normal (less than 5.7 percent), border-line or prediabetes (5.7 to 6.4 percent), or diabetes (6.5 percent or more). It is also possible to test people for diabetes using the same type of glucose tolerance test that is done during pregnancy. If I am seeing someone after a pregnancy with gestational diabetes, I recommend both tests.

If someone has a normal glucose tolerance test between pregnancies, they still have an increased risk of gestational diabetes in their next pregnancy, but probably less than 50 percent, especially if they didn't need insulin in the previous pregnancy. In this case, in the next pregnancy we would normally screen them twice in pregnancy for gestational diabetes: once around 12 to 16 weeks and then again at the more typical 24 to 28 weeks. Also, I would recommend regular exercise and a healthy diet.

When someone has impaired glucose tolerance between pregnancies, we recommend the same things, though the risk of recurrent gestational diabetes is much higher. As noted at the beginning of this chapter, for someone with overt diabetes, treatment prior to pregnancy is critical. Anyone who has diabetes entering pregnancy will have in-creased screening for fetal anomalies, such as a special ultrasound of the fetal heart called a fetal echocardiogram.

Fortunately, for women without diabetes who develop gestational diabetes, and even for most women with overt diabetes, as long as we can keep glucose levels mostly normal in pregnancy, outcomes are usually excellent for mother and baby.

Bottom Line

- Recurrence risk is high on average, but much higher if you have an elevated glucose test between pregnancies.
- Exercise may lower the risk of recurrence.
- Treatment with diet and insulin is very effective if this condition does recur.
- Testing for glucose tolerance between pregnancies is important to evaluate the possibility of pregestational diabetes.
- If your glucose levels are elevated, your doctor or midwife will want to get them to be normal in pregnancy.
- With normal glucose levels, risks to mom and baby are low.

CHAPTER 8

Preeclampsia

DEFINITION: A condition in pregnancy or postpartum characterized by high blood pressure, protein in urine, and sometimes more serious complications

OVERALL PREVALENCE: About 5 percent

RECURRENCE RISK GROUP: Intermediate (20 to 50 percent)

Preeclampsia is a condition that manifests typically toward the end of pregnancy or postpartum and is characterized by a new onset of high blood pressure (hypertension). It is typically marked by protein in the urine (which is a sign of the condition but is in itself harmless). Most women are tested for this frequently throughout pregnancy—it's why they take your blood pressure and have you pee in a cup at each visit.

Preeclampsia is moderately common (about 5 percent of pregnancies are affected). The risk is higher for older women, for women carrying multiple pregnancies, for women with obesity, and for those with hypertension before pregnancy.

A central feature of preeclampsia is that the severity varies tremendously. To give a general overview, preeclampsia is divided into five levels of severity.

- *Gestational hypertension.* Mild elevation of blood pressure starting after 20 weeks (140/90 or greater, but not as high as 160/110), with no other signs or symptoms. If you have hypertension prior to 20 weeks, it is most likely chronic hypertension and not a complication of pregnancy.
- *Preeclampsia, mild.* Mild elevation of blood pressure starting after 20 weeks plus protein in the urine above a certain threshold. There is not much clinical difference between mild gestational hypertension and mild preeclampsia, and the treatment is the same.
- *Preeclampsia, severe.* Gestational hypertension or preeclampsia with any of the following severe features: severe hypertension (160/110 or higher), elevated liver enzymes, low platelets, kidney dysfunction, symptoms suggestive of neurologic dysfunction (severe headache, visual impairment), fluid in the lungs. Often there is fetal growth restriction, but this is no longer a criterion to diagnose severe disease.
- *HELLP.* An acronym for a form of severe preeclampsia when the blood tests show *h*emolysis, *e*levated *l*iver enzymes, and *l*ow *p*latelets. Technically, the blood pressure does not even need to be elevated.
- *Eclampsia.* Preeclampsia followed by a seizure specific to this condition.

The more severe the case, the more complicated the outcomes and choices that families face. Put simply: the only cure for preeclampsia is delivery. And this generates an inherent conflict. The health of the mother is protected by the delivery, but the health of the baby may be compromised.

When preeclampsia develops at or close to full term, then the baby is usually delivered immediately and there is typically little trade-off.

When the condition develops earlier in pregnancy, there is a complex balance between the health of the mother and the health of the baby. This can be a challenging situation, both medically and emotionally. Pregnancies with preeclampsia are often also complicated by preterm birth, a cesarean section, and other issues.

When families move to considering another pregnancy, these complications—and the trade-offs between mother and baby—are often on their mind. As one woman told me:

• • •

Preeclampsia led to a 34-week delivery, plus the baby had major medical complications (stroke). The decision to have another baby took three years plus a lot of therapy. I was scared about delivering early again and something happening to the baby. We almost didn't have another. But after talking with Stanford high-risk OBs and figuring out what another pregnancy would be like (high-risk), we did it. She was born just three weeks ago. I did get hypertension, but we were able to wait and deliver at 37 weeks.

• • •

Or, from another perspective:

• • •

Our daughter spent a month in the NICU following her birth. It feels self-
ish to subject a future child to the same experience our daughter had.

• • •

At the same time, many families I talked to badly wanted their
child to have a sibling, or felt that their family was not yet complete.
For this reason, questions related to recurrence and treatment here
are always top of mind.

WHAT THE DATA SAYS: RECURRENCE AND TREATMENT

Recurrence

In general, it is widely accepted that preeclampsia in one pregnancy is
a risk factor for future pregnancies. The key question is: How high is
that risk?

There are numerous studies on the risk of preeclampsia recurrence.
This is true for a couple of reasons. One is that preeclampsia is relatively
common and it is serious, so it's a focus for many doctors. As important
is the fact—discussed more shortly—that we have at least some evidence that treatment with aspirin early in pregnancy may lower the risk
of developing the condition. Given the potential for treatment, it is especially important to evaluate the risk factors for developing it.

A 2016 article in the *British Medical Journal* (*BMJ*) provides a

comprehensive look.[1] The authors review a total of ninety-two studies, covering more than 25 million pregnancies, to evaluate what factors raise the risk of preeclampsia. Many of these studies consider
prior preeclampsia in their risk factors, and they are able to rely on
data on about 3.7 million women in many countries for this question.

Overall, they find that the risk without prior preeclampsia is about 3
percent, versus 16 percent for women with a history. As we've seen with
other complications, the increase seems to be even larger for women
who had severe cases. Two studies of recurrence risk among women
with severe preeclampsia in an earlier pregnancy put the risk at 47 percent and 65 percent for recurrence. Prior preeclampsia is not the only
predictive risk factor in the model, but it has the highest relative risk.

To summarize, here are the approximate recurrence risks for preeclampsia, based on the previous pregnancy:

First Pregnancy Outcome	Approximate Risk of Preeclampsia in Second Pregnancy
No preeclampsia	1–5%
Mild preeclampsia at term	10%, usually mild preeclampsia at term
Mild preeclampsia preterm (< [as later] 37 weeks)	15%–20%, ranges in severity and timing
Severe preeclampsia or HELLP at term	15%–20%, ranges in severity and timing
Severe preeclampsia or HELLP preterm (< [as later] 37 weeks)	50%, usually severe or preterm, or both

In addition to prior preeclampsia and severity, there are other
demographic factors that contribute to risk. Online, at the Fetal

Medicine Foundation, you can find a calculator that allows you to input detailed information about your pregnancy and prior history to calculate a personal risk.[2]

We've already highlighted the correlation between complications during pregnancy and health outcomes later in life. In this case, anyone with a history of preeclampsia has an increased risk of developing hypertension and heart disease in their lifetime. If you have a history of preeclampsia, make sure that all of your medical providers are made aware, not just your obstetrician.

Treatment

Significant amounts of randomized trial evidence indicate that daily aspirin in pregnancy treatment decreases the risk of preeclampsia. A 2019 Cochrane Review summarizes 72 randomized trials that include almost 40,000 women[3] and concludes that 50 to 150 milligrams daily reduces preeclampsia recurrence risk from about 20 to 16 percent. This treatment is generally started sometime between 12 and 16 weeks. (Quick note: Cochrane Reviews are review articles focused on randomized trials and considered a gold standard approach to combining data from multiple trials.)

Other studies have raised concerns about aspirin in pregnancy, linking it to bleeding during birth. However, these risks are thought to be small and the link tenuous. And longer-term follow-up on at least five thousand children in these trials shows no developmental risks. Low-dose aspirin as prescribed for preeclampsia is considered safe in pregnancy.

Because of the strong evidence for efficacy and the safety evidence, low-dose aspirin is increasingly prescribed even for people who are at only slightly elevated risk for preeclampsia (for example, people who are over a certain age).

The other significant intervention in a later pregnancy is increased monitoring. Home blood-pressure testing or more frequent prenatal visits, for example, can allow for earlier detection of gestational hypertension and preeclampsia. Monitoring leads to better management and, also, if an early delivery is needed, allows for advanced preparation (steroids for lung development, transfer to a hospital with a more advanced NICU).

There are a small number of other interventions with some evidence in their favor. One is calcium supplementation. For people with insufficient calcium intake, supplementation may lower preeclampsia risk.[4] This is a bigger concern in developing countries than in the US or Europe. There isn't strong evidence of a preventive value for women with adequate calcium levels at baseline. However, it is important to note that "adequate" calcium intake is usually defined as 1,000 milligrams a day, which is not typical for most people's diets (a glass of milk has about 300 milligrams of calcium and a serving of yogurt has about 200 milligrams).

There is some, more limited, evidence that weight loss between pregnancies and exercise lowers the risk of preeclampsia. The weight loss evidence is from cohort studies, not randomized trials, and the exercise evidence is from small samples. So while both activities might be a good idea for other reasons, they're not clearly key here.

Unfortunately, many of the interventions that online outlets suggest for preeclampsia—vitamin supplements, changes in diet, fish oil—do not have strong support in the data.

A final note: in 2023 the FDA approved a blood test designed to predict development of preeclampsia among the set of women who are hospitalized with high blood pressure during pregnancy. Although this test isn't used before hypertension has developed, it's an important new diagnosis tool. Continuing research on other possible avenues for both treatment and prevention means that this space is likely to continue to evolve over time.

MEDICAL PERSPECTIVE

Preeclampsia is a condition that can range in severity from a minor annoyance to a life-threatening disease, which is part of the reason it can be difficult to manage, and also why having a prior pregnancy with preeclampsia can mean vastly different things to different people. For some, it was so mild they forgot they even had it, but for others it was a monthlong hospitalization leading to a premature birth followed by two months of hypertension after delivery. On top of that, when it is severe and the pregnancy is preterm, every day brings about a reckoning whether we need to deliver the baby prematurely in order to help the mother's condition improve.

It is crucial to start by establishing the details of the condition in the first pregnancy: When did the preeclampsia begin? How severe was it? Were there any other complications? In part 1 of this book, when we talked about prep work, we emphasized the value of getting access to your medical records. This is a strong example of a condition for which those records would be extremely useful in decision making.

We screen for preeclampsia at every prenatal visit. There are two reasons for this: first, it can happen to anyone without warning, and second, it often has no symptoms until later stages. The most common early symptom is edema (swelling, especially in the legs), but more than 50 percent of women experience this, and only a small fraction of them have preeclampsia.

For most people with a history of preeclampsia, we generally recommend four things. The first two are reflective of the data we've discussed; the other two are a focus on greater monitoring.

1. *Aspirin.* In the US, low-dose aspirin is sold as 81-milligram tablets, nothing else. The safety data for this dose is also very strong, so this is the dose most US women are recommended to take. There is some evidence that 150 milligrams is more effective, so for certain, very high-risk women, I might recommend two baby aspirin (162 milligrams) daily.

2. *Calcium.* As Emily noted, the data on this is mixed. However, the recommended daily intake of calcium for all pregnant women (all women, actually) is 1,000 milligrams a day, so I always ask women if they get that much between their typical diet and their prenatal vitamin. If not, I suggest they take a supplement to get over 1,000 milligrams a day, especially for women at increased risk of preeclampsia. In my experience, most US women do not consume 1,000 milligrams of calcium a day due to low-dairy diets and the low amount of calcium in a typical prenatal vitamin. (Calcium takes up a lot of room. You think your prenatal vitamin is large? Try adding 1,000 milligrams of calcium to it—you might need a fork and knife!)

3. *Home blood-pressure monitoring.* I recommend this routinely to nearly all women with a history of preeclampsia. Home blood-pressure cuffs are automated, easy to use, pretty accurate, and inexpensive. The results can be brought to prenatal visits, sent

in electronically, or even monitored by a remote monitoring system. The biggest advantage to home blood-pressure monitoring is the early identification of hypertension and preeclampsia. Most women will have no symptoms whatsoever when their blood pressure initially goes up, so there is no way to know other than going to the doctor's office. Sure, we see people frequently in pregnancy, but not daily. Unless the blood-pressure cuff is inaccurate, there is really no downside to checking blood pressure at home. Additionally, some women find that their blood pressure is elevated at the doctor's office but not at home (sometimes called white coat hypertension, which is a misnomer—I don't wear a white coat and many of my patients still have it!). This is generally a benign condition and requires no treatment. Without the knowledge that the blood-pressure readings are normal at home, these women might be incorrectly diagnosed with preeclampsia.

I recommend that women with a history of preeclampsia start home blood-pressure monitoring sometime in the third trimester, at least a few weeks before the preeclampsia presented in the prior pregnancy. It should be done once daily (maybe twice; more is usually unnecessary) and should be done at rest and in a seated position. I find the easiest way for women to achieve this is to take it right when they wake up in the morning. Sit up in bed for a minute or two, take the blood pressure, write the number down, and, if it's normal, you're good until tomorrow. Normal is less than 140/90. If it is elevated, take it again and let us know.

4. *Fetal growth assessments.* Women with a history of preeclampsia not only have an increased risk of preeclampsia in the next pregnancy but also have an increased risk of other placenta-mediated

conditions, most notably fetal growth restriction. We don't understand exactly why, but the hypothesis is that preeclampsia and fetal growth restriction are both manifestations of the same problem: an abnormal placenta. So if you have one condition, you are at increased risk for the other. Also, if you have a history of one, you have an increased risk of both in the next pregnancy. For this reason, in women with a prior pregnancy complicated by preeclampsia, I follow up with fetal growth assessments, which means a few extra ultrasounds.

For women with a history of severe preeclampsia requiring delivery prior to 34 weeks, we check bloodwork to test them for antiphospholipid antibody syndrome (an autoimmune condition that occurs in approximately 1 in 2,000 people but is more common in women of reproductive age). If they have this condition, we also treat them with heparin or low-molecular-weight heparin in the next pregnancy.

If you had preeclampsia in a prior pregnancy, there is a very good chance that the aforementioned treatments can improve outcomes in this pregnancy. This can mean preventing preeclampsia entirely or perhaps just making it less severe than in the last pregnancy, or recur at a later gestational age than it presented last time. Even if it does recur exactly the same way as last time, knowing that it may be coming, understanding what to expect, and early detection with home blood-pressure monitoring and close follow-up can lead to improved outcomes for you and your baby, as well as make the experience a little less scary.

Bottom Line

- Recurrence risk of preeclampsia overall is less than 50 percent, but this recurrence is more likely if the condition was more severe in the first pregnancy.
- Treatment with baby aspirin reduces the risk of recurrence by about 20 percent.
- Supplementation with calcium may be effective if you are calcium deficient.
- Get detailed medical records: the specifics of your case are important.
- The main treatments to prevent recurrence or lessen the severity are low-dose aspirin, calcium, home blood-pressure monitoring, and fetal testing.
- If you had severe preeclampsia prior to 34 weeks, you should be tested for antiphospholipid antibody syndrome.

~~~~~~~~~

CHAPTER 9

Fetal Growth Restriction

DEFINITIONS:

SMALL FOR GESTATIONAL AGE (SGA): Infant or fetus that is small relative to gestational age (under the 10th percentile)

FETAL GROWTH RESTRICTION (FGR): Infant or fetus that is small due to a medical problem

OVERALL PREVALENCE:

SGA: By definition, about 10 percent of babies or fetuses

FGR: A subset of the babies/fetuses with SGA (so, less than 10 percent)

RECURRENCE RISK GROUP: Intermediate (10 to 50 percent)

This chapter focuses on fetal growth restriction (FGR), but it's useful to start by talking about a related, but more common, diagnosis: small for gestational age (SGA).

SGA is a broad diagnosis that is usually defined as *below the 10th percentile for a given gestational age at birth*. A diagnosis of SGA is straightforward and mechanical: if a baby's weight or fetus's estimated weight is below the 10th percentile, then there is SGA. As a result, about 10 percent of babies will be SGA, and for the most part they just represent one end of the normal distribution of human size.

On its own, SGA is not necessarily a concern. However, in some cases, a fetus that is SGA can be a result of fetal growth restriction (FGR) or intrauterine growth restriction (IUGR). These diagnoses are more concerning, as they reflect situations in which a baby or fetus was supposed to be bigger, but some problem led to them being smaller. Growth restriction can be caused by a wide variety of problems, including poor placental function, malnutrition, maternal disease, infections, exposures (like smoking), and genetic abnormalities.

In practice, these terms—SGA, FGR, and IUGR—are sometimes used interchangeably. A fetus that is SGA is likely to be suspected to have FGR, even if in most cases they do not. In practice, a fetus measuring under the 10th percentile for weight should be considered SGA and "possible" or "suspected" FGR.

I start with this somewhat technical context here because it matters quite a lot for thinking about recurrence and, more importantly, the risk of adverse and long-term complications. Notably, if we think SGA is just a result of normal variation, then while there is a significant recurrence risk (first baby weight is predictive of later baby weight, for a variety of reasons), it's less likely to be a *concern*. If the reason for the SGA is because of a growth restriction, this is of more concern and a case in which more attention will be paid to prevention.

While the distinction between SGA and FGR is important for thinking about possible treatment, it is not always an easy one to make in practice. As a general rule, the smaller the baby is, the more doctors will worry that FGR is playing a role. In line with this, the smaller the baby, the higher the risk of complications.

WHAT THE DATA SAYS: RECURRENCE AND PREVENTION

Recurrence

Having had a first baby diagnosed with SGA increases the risk in future pregnancies. Data from almost 13,000 women in the Netherlands provides us with a significant number of first-pregnancy SGA diagnoses (the smallest 5 percent of babies was their threshold for diagnosis).[1] Among those women, 23 percent received the same diagnosis in a second pregnancy, while only 3.4 percent of second pregnancies without a first-pregnancy diagnosis fell within SGA range. Data from over 300,000 women in the US shows a similar correlation—24 percent of women with SGA in a first pregnancy had it in a second, versus only 6 percent of those without.[2]

SGA in a first pregnancy has also been associated with other risks in later pregnancies, notably stillbirth. In a large sample of 400,000 Swedish women, researchers found that, compared with women whose first birth was full term and not SGA, those with a full-term SGA birth were twice as likely to have a stillbirth in a subsequent pregnancy.[3] The risk was five times as high if the prior birth was both SGA and very preterm (less than 32 weeks' gestation). It isn't clear why this is; it may well reflect a more significant problem in the first pregnancy that led to a small baby and preterm birth, such as a placental disorder.

Prevention

Lowering the risk of SGA in a later pregnancy is somewhat dependent on whether the cause is known. For example, SGA can sometimes be a result of preeclampsia. If that's the case, then treatment with aspirin, which would lower the risk of recurrent preeclampsia, can help here, too. SGA is also more common for women who smoke. Quitting smoking in a later pregnancy would lower the risk.

However, in many cases, the underlying cause of an SGA diagnosis isn't clear. This makes it much more difficult to know how to lower the risk.

One behavioral approach that may play a role is avoiding a short interval between pregnancies; even outside those with a history of SGA, a short interval (especially less than three months) between pregnancies is associated with a higher risk of SGA than a longer interval.[4]

A second approach may be encouraging more weight gain. There is a link between weight gain and fetal size, with more maternal weight gain (on average) being associated with larger babies. These effects are consistent, although relatively small—in one study, two groups were compared in which one gained an average of 17 pounds more during pregnancy.[5] The authors found the babies in the higher weight gain group were an average of about 0.6 pounds larger.

The question of whether weight gain should be encouraged is a complicated one. Despite the correlation, it's not obvious whether more weight gain will actually lead to a larger baby. And, beyond this, it's unclear in these cases whether having a larger baby will actually generate any health benefits.

On the flip side, there are a number of interventions that have been tried but do not seem to work. They include blood thinners, bed rest, fatty-acid supplementation, and antihypertensive drugs. One trial, published in 2021, suggested a positive impact of stress reduction or a Mediterranean diet on the risk of SGA.[6] However, there are some technical issues that render the study at least in need of replication before universal adoption. Meditating and consuming more olive oil may be good for other reasons! It is just not clear that it helps here.

Additional monitoring should certainly be a part of later pregnancies after growth restriction. This is especially true given the link with higher stillbirth risk. Monitoring with ultrasounds, nonstress tests, and more frequent prenatal visits will allow for possible earlier detection of complications. It may also allow for better understanding of the scope of the problem. Some fetuses are just small but growing on a steady trajectory. This is much less concerning than a fetus that is not growing steadily. Repeated ultrasounds for size can help to better clarify the situation.

MEDICAL PERSPECTIVE

As Emily noted, if the definition of SGA is simply a baby measuring less than the 10th percentile for weight, then also by definition 10 percent of babies born will have SGA. So, as you may imagine, I see a lot of patients with a history of SGA! When I am speaking with people about SGA, I usually break it down into the following categories:

1. *There is no problem.* This is by far the most common "cause" of SGA—the baby is just small. Like adults, there is a wide range of normal sizes for babies. Some babies are long (since they don't

stand up, we call them long, not tall), some are short, some are heavy, some are thin, etc. This is sometimes also called constitutional delay (a great example of a term that is not helpful for doctors or patients).

2. *There is a problem with the placenta.* This is also called placental insufficiency. In this situation, the baby is "supposed" to be bigger, but for some reason the placenta is doing a poor job of transferring calories and nutrients from the mother to the fetus.

In the setting of SGA, I will usually suspect the placenta is the problem if there are other features on ultrasound that also point in that direction, like low amniotic fluid or abnormal blood flow in the umbilical cord. Also, there are certain conditions in the mother that make this more likely, such as high blood pressure or diabetes. Finally, if the baby has a very small abdomen (i.e., the baby is very skinny), the placenta is more likely to be the problem. This makes sense, as a lack of calories from the placenta is more likely to cause a fetus to be skinny rather than have a small head size, just like it would for a child or adult. This is sometimes called asymmetric growth restriction.

3. *There is a problem with the fetus.* This could be due to a genetic abnormality, an infection, or an exposure to a toxin (like smoking). We suspect this when there are other ultrasound features of a fetal abnormality. It is the reason we frequently recommend genetic and infectious testing of small babies. This is done in pregnancy with amniocentesis or after birth with a blood test.

4. *There is a problem with the mother.* Malnutrition is an example, and it is fortunately pretty rare in developed countries. Other serious maternal chronic illnesses can cause growth restriction, but they are usually known prior to the pregnancy. The one ex-

ception is antiphospholipid antibody syndrome, which can be silent or a recently acquired condition and can present for the first time with severe fetal growth restriction.

Based on the cause of the SGA in the first pregnancy, or the most likely cause, it is a little easier to predict the risk of recurrence. If we think the baby was small just due to variation in size (reason 1), then there is a high chance of recurrence (25 to 50 percent or higher), because children with similar genetics tend to be similar sizes. However, even though it is likely to recur, it isn't likely to be a *problem*, because it was never a problem. Problems with the placenta are most often sporadic, and the recurrence risk is lower, probably closer to 20 percent, based on my experience. Genetic and infectious causes tend to be nearly entirely sporadic, and the recurrence risk is very small. If the cause was a severe maternal condition, such as uncontrolled hypertension, the recurrence risk would depend on whether the condition is the same, better, or worse in the next pregnancy.

One notable exception is severe early-onset growth restriction due to antiphospholipid antibody syndrome, an autoimmune condition that is rare but more common in women of reproductive age and can contribute to a variety of pregnancy complications. If this test is positive, it is treated with low-dose aspirin and injectable anticoagulants, such as heparin. Without treatment, the recurrence risk is very high. With treatment, it is much lower.

If this test is negative, the cause is likely a very unhealthy placenta, which is often sporadic, or a fetal genetic or infectious cause, which are also sporadic. Therefore, this is one situation where those with the absolute worst first outcome tend to have a good outcome the next time around.

Here is a summary table:

Cause of SGA	Recurrence Risk	Notes
There is no problem (baby was just small)	25–50%	When it recurs, also likely not a problem
Placental insufficiency	Approximately 20%	
Genetic / infections	Less than 5%	
Maternal condition	Depends on the condition and if it improved between pregnancies	
Antiphospholipid antibody syndrome	Greater than 50%	With treatment, probably closer to 20%

In practice, we often do not know the cause of the SGA. Therefore, we usually do serial growth measurements in the subsequent pregnancy for everyone with a prior SGA newborn. If there is once again SGA during pregnancy, we will typically recommend more testing to help assess the cause again. This includes more frequent ultrasounds, nonstress tests or biophysical profiles, and sometimes bloodwork and potentially an amniocentesis.

If you had a prior SGA baby, it makes sense to follow up in the next pregnancy, at least for your ultrasounds, with a doctor who has a lot of experience with this condition. Having a strong understanding of SGA can often be helpful in reducing stress and anxiety for you in the next pregnancy, as the additional testing will be more standard practice for us and our experience would suggest that we can be relatively confident that with close monitoring, the baby will likely be fine.

Bottom Line

- In the majority of cases in which a baby is small for gestational age, they are *not* growth restricted, and there is nothing pathological or problematic.
- If fetal growth restriction was suspected in a previous pregnancy, treatment will depend on the cause.
- Avoiding short pregnancy intervals and trying to gain more weight may be positive changes.
- Expect to have more frequent ultrasounds to monitor growth in the next pregnancy.

CHAPTER 10

Preterm Birth

DEFINITION: Birth before 37 completed weeks of gestation

OVERALL PREVALENCE: In the US, 10.5 percent of all births

RECURRENCE RISK GROUP: Intermediate (15 to 30 percent)

Although the vast majority of preterm infants survive, prematurity is still the leading cause of infant mortality in the US and also a significant cause of developmental disabilities, both physical and intellectual. Preterm birth is a complication experienced unequally across groups; the preterm birth rate is about 14 percent among Black women versus 9 percent among white women. It is one significant reason for worse health outcomes for Black infants.

Preterm birth can be "indicated," meaning that it occurs as a response to some other complication (preeclampsia, for example). In these cases, the underlying concern is with the initial complication and so in subsequent pregnancies, you and your doctor will take proactive steps to address them. Preterm birth can also be "spontane-ous," meaning it occurs without seeming to be prompted by another complication. We will focus on those cases in this chapter.

The definition of preterm birth as birth before 37 weeks of com-pleted gestation cannot capture the vast variation within the group of preterm births. Babies born as early as 23 weeks of gestation can sur-vive. But the experience of having a child born at 36 weeks and one born at 24 weeks is likely to be completely different.

The starkest way to see this in the data is through mortality risk. The graph on the next page shows the share of births by week, as well as the mortality risk for these births. Only 0.1 percent of births occur at 23 weeks of gestation, and only about a third of those infants sur-vive. In contrast, 4.49 percent of births occur at 36 weeks, close to full term, and survival in that group is 99 percent, close to the overall fig-ure for full-term infants (99.5 percent).[1]

We can also see these differences in how women describe their ex-periences. I contrast the two below—one from someone who gave birth around 25 weeks, and the other around 36 weeks.

• • •

Our second child was born at 24 weeks, five days, weighing just over 700 grams. She spent 145 days in the intensive care nursery, with her most long-term complication being a total colectomy (removal of colon) due to necrotizing enterocolitis. Aside from the trauma, a lengthy NICU stay, and bringing home a medically complicated child, I was also recovering from a classical (vertical incision) C-section. It took us five years to decide to try for another pregnancy.

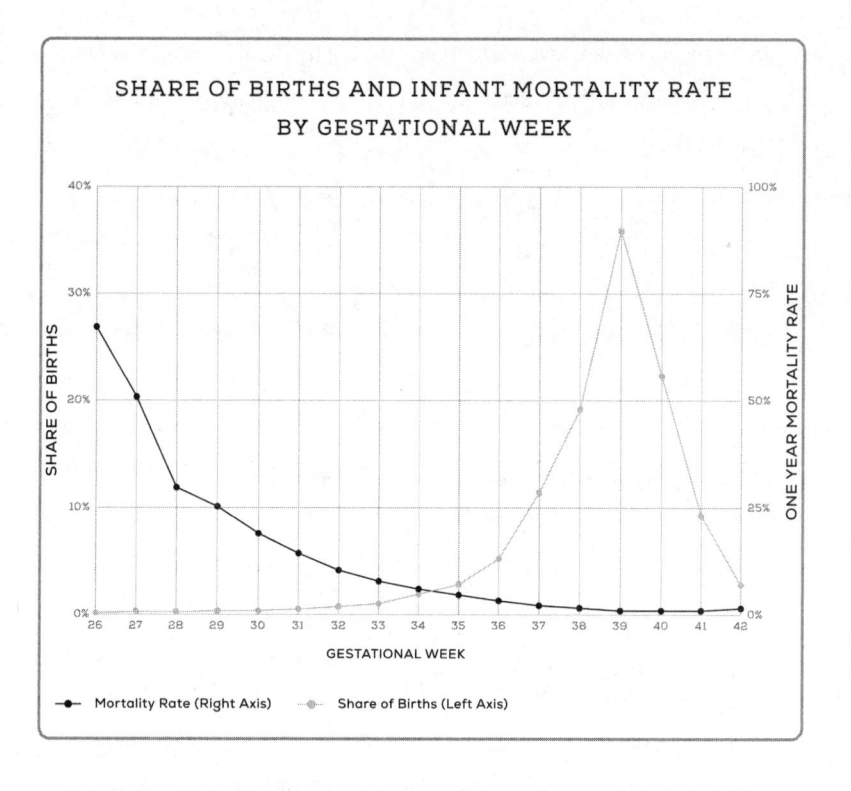

SHARE OF BIRTHS AND INFANT MORTALITY RATE
BY GESTATIONAL WEEK

I gave birth at 36 weeks. While our baby is healthy, the birth itself was an uncomplicated vaginal delivery, and our baby did not need a NICU stay, the experience of having a premature baby who we had to care for alone at home was incredibly difficult, and very different than the experiences of anyone else in my network, who largely had full-term babies or premature babies who stayed in the NICU until they were term. The four extra newborn weeks and the special feeding schedule we did for that time were grueling. My husband's paternity leave ended before we even made it to the expected due date. I still feel jealous of the experience of friends with

full-term births and have a hard time listening to friends complain about
the discomforts of being eight and nine months pregnant, when I never
made it that far.

. . .

What strikes me here, in reading these, is that while the *experiences*
these two women had were extremely different, the feeling of trauma
is not. Preterm birth, especially when it is not for a known reason, is
unexpected and frightening. Everything is going well, and then, all of
a sudden, it isn't. One woman captured it well:

. . .

My son was born at 28 weeks, zero days gestational age. I noticed a slow-
down in movement and went to the hospital to get checked out. I figured
they'd send me home in an hour with some reassurance and a lollipop.
They did not. Twelve hours later, after a flurry of stops and starts, our
son was born via emergency C-section. He spent 10 weeks in the NICU
with breathing support, brain bleeding and swelling, and more. And
against all odds, he is now a healthy 3-year-old with no lasting implica-
tions from his early arrival.

. . .

The consequence of all this, when you think about trying to get
pregnant again, is often anxiety. Among women who have had a preterm birth, many talk about the significant anxiety associated with a
later pregnancy—or even the contemplation of a later pregnancy.

• • •

My anxiety made me have biweekly check-ins with my doctor.

• • •

Mentally, it has been challenging. Even when the data is clear, when you've been the outlier, it is hard to believe the odds.

• • •

I had originally considered trying for a second child, but I don't know if we can go through that again.

• • •

Alleviating that anxiety is a huge, and probably insurmountable, challenge. But the data can offer some clarity to the anxiety-provoking questions of "Will it happen again?" and "Can I prevent it?" No matter how well-informed you are, though, anxiety may be inevitable. Finding ways to support yourself through that should be part of your preparation.

So if you had a prior preterm birth, it is important to investigate why it happened and what might be helpful to prevent it, or improve outcomes, in a subsequent pregnancy. But it is equally important to remember that most people with a preterm birth do not have one in a subsequent pregnancy, or have a less preterm birth, either because the reason for the preterm birth was a onetime event or because the treatments we have are effective. Aim to strike a fair balance between vigilance and optimism.

The same applies to your doctors—it is important to find someone with a lot of experience with preterm birth so she or he can also provide that balance.

WHAT THE DATA SAYS:
RECURRENCE AND PREVENTION

Recurrence

First, a preterm birth in one pregnancy does increase the risk of prematurity in later pregnancies. But by how much?

The largest datasets on this question come out of Europe. In Denmark, researchers used data on 536,000 women who had two singleton deliveries over the period from 1978 through 2007.[2] They found that for women who had a first birth at full term (37 weeks or more), only 2.7 percent of them had a preterm delivery in their second pregnancy. This number was 14.7 percent for women who delivered between 32 and 36 weeks, 25.4 percent for those who delivered between 28 and 32 weeks, and 26 percent for those who delivered before 28 weeks in their first pregnancy.

A similar paper with data out of Japan echoed these results: 16 percent of women with a prior preterm delivery had a recurrence.[3] A study of about 50,000 women in Utah suggested slightly higher numbers: a 30 percent risk of preterm birth recurrence in a second pregnancy.[4] A survey of 1,700 women at multiple study sites in the US, run by the National Institute of Child Health and Human Development, showed a risk of about 22 percent, versus 9 percent in pregnancies to women with no prior preterm birth.[5]

So we can see that the risks here are substantially elevated, though notably not to 100 percent. Using the Danish data, among women whose first birth was prior to 28 weeks, about 75 percent of them did *not* have a preterm delivery in their second birth. The most important variable here seems to be the degree of preterm birth: the earlier the first birth, the more likely that later births will be at least somewhat preterm.

The risks of recurrent preterm birth also are higher for women with a shorter interval between pregnancies.[6] In the data, having less than six months between giving birth and being pregnant again does seem to increase the risk of a second preterm birth. It is not clear why this would be, and it is also not clear that the relationship here is *causal*. There are other factors that are linked to closely spaced pregnancies, some of which themselves seem to increase the risk of preterm birth. When researchers adjust for those factors, the link between birth spacing and preterm birth is weaker.[7]

In some cases, there is an obvious explanation. If the cause was an infection, then this is unlikely to recur. If the first birth was twins, a subsequent singleton pregnancy does not seem to have an elevated preterm birth risk.[8]

Prevention

Preparation

In the first part of this book, I talked about framing preparation as a type of treatment. Being associated with a hospital with better capacity, or having more frequent check-ins, can allow you to reach a better outcome. This is especially true with preterm birth, where treatment with steroids can improve lung development.[9] While I won't revisit this discussion here, I want to acknowledge again that even if the same challenges arise, preparation alone can make the experience very different.

Progesterone

The most commonly discussed and prescribed treatment for preterm birth is progesterone supplements, either in the form of injections or vaginal suppositories. Broadly, the reasoning behind this is that progesterone produced internally is important for maintaining pregnancy in several ways (hence the name progesterone: *pro* [in favor of], *gest* [pregnancy, like *gestation*], *erone* [the type of compound it is]). In theory, then, external progesterone could also contribute.

This treatment could be appropriate for preterm birth even if the cause is unknown—effectively, the first category I discussed earlier, where preterm birth simply happens without warning or an obvious explanation.

Whether this works in practice is subject to significant debate. This debate has been most active in recent years around the injectable form of progesterone—17-hydroxyprogesterone caproate, or 17-OHPC or 17P—which was marketed as the drug Makena. A little background: progesterone was used since the 1970s to reduce the risk of preterm birth, but it became the standard of care after a large randomized trial was published in 2003 in the *New England Journal of Medicine*.[10]

The trial enrolled 463 women who had a prior preterm birth and were pregnant again. They were randomized into treatment or control. The treatment group was given weekly injections of progesterone starting sometime between 16 and 20 weeks and going through 36 weeks of pregnancy. The authors found a 34 percent reduction in the risk of birth before 37 weeks of pregnancy and a 42 percent reduction in the risk of delivery before 32 weeks. These effects are large. The infants born to treatment mothers—as a result of being less likely to be born preterm—were also less likely to suffer complications.

Despite these promising results, prior to 2011 this drug wasn't FDA-approved and prescriptions needed to go through compounding pharmacies (pharmacies that mix the approved ingredients themselves and make the drug), making them difficult to access. Some doctors, pharmacists, and patients were understandably apprehensive about using a non-FDA-approved medication in this way.

In 2011 the FDA approved a standard form of this injectable under the name Makena. This wasn't a new drug—Makena is the same product that was being produced by the compounding pharmacies—but by approving the standard formulation, the hope was that it would be more widely accessible and safe. Importantly, by approving it this way, the FDA gave Makena a monopoly on the drug, meaning it couldn't be accessed through the compounding pharmacies except as an "off-label" medication.

However, follow-up research has called into question the efficacy of progesterone treatment. FDA approval of the drug was based on the original randomized trial in 2003. When approving the medication, the FDA required the drug company to fund a second, larger study on efficacy. That was published in 2020.[11]

This second study enrolled about 1,700 women at 93 clinical centers worldwide and randomized them into treatment with the drug or a control. It did not find any impact of the drug on preterm birth rates. The rate of preterm birth before 35 weeks was 11 percent in the treatment group and 11.5 percent in the placebo. These were not significantly different, and the authors didn't find any other notable differences across groups, either.

This study is much larger than the original, but it is not without its own problems. The population of people turned out to be at lower risk for preterm birth. In the original study, over 50 percent of the control group had a preterm birth. In the follow-up, the rate was 11.5 percent. That makes it much harder to pick up impacts and suggests that the results might not generalize to a high-risk population of women.

This whole messy debate left the FDA in the awkward position of having approved a drug with seemingly little benefit (it was also very expensive). In response, the FDA's Center for Drug Evaluation and Research suggested that the Makena approval be withdrawn, which occurred in October 2022. Although 17-OHPC is still available, it is now prescribed to compounding pharmacies, which prepare the medication themselves (similar to how it was done before Makena was marketed).

Adding to the confusion, a 2021 meta-analysis of *all* studies of both vaginal and injectable forms of progesterone was slightly more positive.[12] That meta-analysis showed that vaginal progesterone decreased the risk of birth before 34 weeks by about 20 percent and showed a similar impact with 17-OHPC, though one that just slightly misses statistical significance. That study also found some improvements in infant health at birth (i.e., less NICU time, less need for respiratory support) with the vaginal suppositories.

Given the mixed evidence on benefits, an obvious follow-up question is whether there are significant risks to this treatment. Based on the recent meta-analysis, any short-term risks appear to be very limited. A 2022 study of children of women exposed to 17-OHPC in utero in the early 1960s looked at the risks of cancer in adulthood and found a slightly elevated risk.[13] This may deserve more study, but at the moment the numbers are extremely small—the study had only 234 exposed women, and the progesterone used, as well as the timing, was different from the formulations used today.

Overall, this is a balance. The potential impacts are small. They may not be zero, but the drug certainly isn't a panacea. It's a clear case where joint decision making is key. Generally, the higher the risk of recurrent preterm birth (such as a prior preterm birth at a very early gestational age, or several preterm births), the more likely progesterone will be helpful. As for the formulation of progesterone, 17-OHPC or vaginal, current recommendations are not to use 17P and to (maybe) use vaginal progesterone, but these decisions often come down to availability, cost, and patient preference. This is also something that will likely evolve over time (and this book will evolve with it).

Cerclage

A second standard treatment for preventing preterm birth recurrence is cerclage, which addresses preterm birth as the result of a physical problem with the cervix rather than a hormonal one. This is a procedure in which a suture (stitch) is placed around the cervix to prevent it from dilating too soon. The stitch would generally be placed between 12 and 24 weeks of pregnancy and then removed close to term. The operation is done by an OB-GYN or MFM.

Cerclage is an old, well-known treatment but there is no large-scale randomized trial evidence for its efficacy. Case reports, observational studies, expert opinion, and biological plausibility are the most important arguments for its usage. There are a number of small randomized trials that, combined, yield data on about 3,500 women. A Cochrane Review of these data published in 2017 showed a reduction of about 23 percent in preterm birth as a result of cerclage.[14] Given the relatively small samples, the researchers cannot rule out the possibility of much smaller or larger effects. This review also includes studies that compare cerclage versus progesterone, but the trials were too small to distinguish between those in any precise way.

From a data standpoint, this is underwhelming. There may be a moderate reduction in the risk of preterm birth after cerclage. Making this more complex, though, is that cerclage is intended to treat a *specific* issue with the cervix, not more generally to treat preterm birth. This suggests a key role for other clinical information. In his section, Nate will talk more about this particular intervention and when it might be most useful to discuss with your provider.

Less Common Prevention Options: Aspirin, Fish Oil, Bacterial Vaginosis Screening

Preterm birth is common, so it is perhaps unsurprising that the medical system explores a wide range of possible treatments.

Aspirin came up in the prevention of preeclampsia in the last chapter, and there is also speculation that it decreases preterm birth. This speculation has been based largely on secondary analyses of data that were designed to evaluate the impact of aspirin in preventing preeclampsia. However, in 2022 a randomized trial including 400 women was published that evaluated the efficacy of aspirin for preventing preterm birth specifically.[15]

This trial, unfortunately, was what we call *underpowered*—there were not enough people in the study to generate statistical precision. The authors found a 23 percent reduction in preterm birth with aspirin usage. But from a statistical standpoint, they could not reject that there was no impact. This isn't encouraging, but it's so imprecise that it is difficult to learn much of anything. Given the impacts of pre-eclampsia and the overall low risks from low-dose aspirin, it seems likely that a large share of women will be prescribed aspirin, just in case. But for stronger evidence that it works, we'll have to wait for a larger trial.

A second treatment that has some positive evidence is increased omega-3 consumption. Omega-3 fatty acids are found at high levels in fish and at lower levels in flax and chia seeds; they can also be taken as supplements. Omega-3s are thought to enhance brain development, so they are a common inclusion in prenatal vitamins.

A 2018 meta-analysis that included 70 randomized controlled trials of almost 20,000 women from a variety of countries found that omega-3 supplementation (either through pills or food) during pregnancy lowered the risk of preterm birth.[16] The reductions were moderate to large: a 10 percent reduction in births before 37 weeks and a 40 percent reduction in births before 34 weeks. Both of these were statistically significant, and the authors also found a statistically significant reduction in the risk of low birth weight, as well as suggestive evidence (with marginal statistical significance) of a lower risk of infant mortality.

There are open questions in the case of omega-3s. What is the right dose? Is it better to get it through food or through supplements? Do some benefit more than others? Despite the questions, there are little or no known downsides to increasing consumption of these products, and, indeed, they are recommended as healthy for other reasons.

Finally, bacterial vaginosis is an overgrowth of bacteria in the vagina found in 10 to 25 percent of pregnant women and has been associated with preterm birth. Screening and treating all pregnant women for bacterial vaginosis to prevent preterm birth has been studied in many prospective trials and does not seem to be effective. Some studies showed benefit to high-risk women, especially those with a history of preterm premature rupture of membranes (water breaking). Certain antibiotics, such as oral clindamycin, seem to be more effective in reducing preterm birth than others, such as metronidazole. Routine screening for bacterial vaginosis is not common, but it may be recommended if you've had a prior preterm birth, accompanied by a course of clindamycin if you test positive.

Preventions with No Evidence: Bed Rest, Uterine Monitoring

There are some commonly prescribed treatments for preterm birth that do not work and, in at least the case of bed rest, can be actively harmful.

Bed rest does not appear to be helpful at decreasing the risks of preterm birth. A 2015 Cochrane Review concludes: "Although bed rest in hospital or at home is widely used as the first step of treatment, there is no evidence that this practice could be beneficial."[17] There are no extremely large randomized trials, so it is difficult to be fully conclusive, but some studies have even found that preterm birth is higher for those on activity restriction.[18]

There is also evidence of other kinds of harm from bed rest: it can increase depression, decrease physical conditioning and muscle tone, and increase the risk of blood clots. Basically, bed rest is a bad idea.

Another common intervention with little support in the data is home uterine monitoring in the third trimester—that is, having people bring home a device that can monitor their uterine contractions and send information to their providers. There are a number of studies of the treatment, but many of them are of poor quality. In a review, when limiting to good-quality studies, this approach leads to more doctor visits but not better outcomes.[19]

In a sense, the good news is that there are interventions that may prevent preterm birth. Choosing from among these options—some of them? All of them? None of them?—is not necessarily straightforward. For those who find themselves in this situation, the key is working through these questions with your provider.

MEDICAL PERSPECTIVE

Since about 10 percent of deliveries are preterm, this is one of the common reasons I might see someone for consultation. The tenor of the conversation usually follows the experience of the preterm birth. For a patient who had an extremely early delivery of a child who did not survive due to prematurity, they are understandably very focused on the risk of preterm birth and terrified that it will happen again. For a patient who had a healthy delivery at 36 weeks, I still want to discuss preterm birth, and sometimes they are surprised that this is a topic to talk about at all.

If you had a preterm birth in a first pregnancy, the first question in contemplating the risks in a second pregnancy is, "Do we know why this happened?" To answer that, we first need to know whether the preterm birth was indicated or spontaneous.

Indicated Preterm Birth

Sometimes preterm birth is indicated for known reasons (preeclampsia, fetal growth restriction, twin pregnancy). For the most part, if you had an indicated preterm birth, our discussion will focus on the underlying cause.

There are a few specific medical conditions that are potential contributing causes to indicated preterm birth. These include chronic hypertension, long-standing diabetes, and lupus. With these conditions, good management of them between pregnancies is usually the best way to reduce the risk of complications in the next pregnancy.

One less common condition that doctors will sometimes consider in cases of indicated preterm birth is antiphospholipid antibody syndrome. This is a relatively rare autoimmune disorder (1 in 2,000 people), but is most common in women of reproductive age. It can lead to blood clots as well as numerous complications of pregnancy such as miscarriage, preeclampsia, fetal growth restriction, and stillbirth. If you delivered preterm for one of these reasons (usually at less than 34 weeks), I will recommend testing for this condition, which entails a few blood tests, repeated 12 weeks apart. If you do have this condition, treatment in the next pregnancy usually involves low-dose aspirin and a form of a blood thinner, such as low-molecular-weight heparin, which is injected (by you; it's not as bad as it sounds) under your skin once or twice a day.

Spontaneous Preterm Birth

Spontaneous preterm birth is complicated because we usually don't know why you went into labor early. This isn't surprising considering we also usually don't know why someone goes into labor at full term. We understand what happens when you go into labor, but we don't understand why it happens to a particular person on a particular day. In some cases, the precipitating event is your water breaking prematurely, but, again, we do not usually know why.

Very generally, there seem to be five pathways that can ultimately lead to water breaking early or early labor.

1. *Premature activation of the hypothalamic-pituitary-adrenal axis.* When you go into labor at term, there is a complicated feedback system between your brain, the baby's brain, and the placenta. Again, we don't know exactly what gets the ball rolling, but when it happens, it is very hard to turn off. The thought is that some women simply have their "labor clock" set to the wrong date, and it's the normal process of labor occurring, just a month or two early.

2. *Infection.* Many preterm births are accompanied by infection, either overt or subclinical. The infection can precede pregnancy or develop during. Sometimes bacteria from the vagina (the vagina is supposed to have bacteria, but it is kept out of the uterus by several defense mechanisms) finds its way into the uterus and causes an inflammatory reaction, leading to labor or to water breaking prematurely.

3. *Bleeding.* If the placenta separates from the uterus prematurely at the end of pregnancy, there is a lot of bleeding and contractions, and we refer to that as a placental abruption. However, there is also a situation where the placenta separates just a tiny bit from the uterus, causing a small amount of bleeding on and off for a large portion of the pregnancy. The chronic bleeding,

sometimes called a chronic abruption, can also cause an inflammatory reaction, leading to preterm labor.

4. *Uterine distention.* If the uterus is stretched beyond normal, such
as with twin or triplet pregnancies, or if there is an abnormally
large amount of amniotic fluid (polyhydramnios), the uterine muscle may reach a point that triggers contraction and labor.

5. *Cervical insufficiency* (formerly called cervical incompetence).
Conceptually, this refers to a situation where the cervix, which
is the lowest part of the uterus, is too weak to sustain a pregnancy, leading to premature shortening and dilation of the cervix, which then leads to a pregnancy loss or a preterm birth. In
practice, this is very difficult to diagnose, because there is no
test (bloodwork, imaging, biopsy) that can be done when you are
not pregnant. Also, in pregnancy, just because a cervix shortens
or dilates does not mean the cervix is weak. This can also be a
response to inflammation, infection, or contractions.

A first step in thinking through treatment in a second pregnancy is
to assess which of these five reasons is the likely cause. Sometimes it
is fairly clear (i.e., if you had twins in the last pregnancy, that was
probably the reason for preterm birth). Other times it's not, and it's
necessary to hold all potential causes as possibilities.

Given our understanding of the causes of preterm birth, when I see
patients with a prior preterm birth, I usually focus on a thorough history and review of records, which may help elucidate the cause of the
preterm birth, as well as the treatments attempted at the time. Based
on the circumstances, I might recommend some tests prior to the next
pregnancy, most commonly an evaluation of the uterine cavity shape
to assess for a uterine abnormality (not common, but important to

know about). This can be done with an ultrasound or an MRI. It is unusual for anything to be found on physical examination that will be helpful, aside, perhaps, from a cervical laceration (tear), which would indicate a cervical problem and the need for cerclage.

I also generally suggest screening for bacterial vaginosis in the next pregnancy, usually in the first or early second trimester. As Emily notes, there is not a huge body of evidence in favor of this, but in practice I often suggest it since the screening and treatment is simple.

After this, there are really two key decisions. The first is whether to use progesterone starting at 16 to 20 weeks, and if so, whether to use 17P injections or vaginal progesterone. Since the data surrounding progesterone are complex, there is a lot of leeway with these decisions. In general, the earlier the preterm birth, the more likely I am going to recommend progesterone and the more likely a patient is going to want to take it. For example, the patient who had a 26-week preterm birth and a baby in the NICU for four months is more likely to be on board for progesterone the next time around than someone who delivered at 36.5 weeks and the baby went home with them the next day. The data supports this as well—the earlier the preterm birth, the more data there are to support progesterone.

As for the type of progesterone, in my practice it comes down to patient preference between an injection once a week and a vaginal suppository once a day. There are sometimes cost or insurance or availability differences as well. Current recommendations favor vaginal progesterone over 17P, but this may evolve over time.

The second decision is about whether to place a cerclage, which is relevant if the cause of preterm birth was cervical insufficiency.

In my view, cerclage is one of the most misunderstood interventions we have in obstetrics. It used to be that all doctors recommended cerclages, then they fell out of favor ("cerclage does not work" was what I was told during my fellowship), and then cerclages made a comeback. One likely reason there has been such flip-flopping on cerclage is that it is so hard to reliably determine whether you actually have cervical insufficiency or not. The more likely it is that a weak cervix is your problem, the more likely a cerclage will be helpful. The less likely that a weak cervix is your problem, the less likely that a cerclage will be helpful and the more likely that it will be harmful. Also, cerclage is not a standardized intervention, like an injection of progesterone. It is a surgical procedure that requires significant skill, and not every doctor has equal skill or technique.

The upshot of this is that cerclage is likely a good idea if a weak cervix is your problem, and not a good idea if it is not your problem. To figure this out, doctors rely on your specific history, what your cervix looks like on ultrasound (if you are pregnant), and how it appears and feels on examination.

In general, cerclage appears to be helpful in the following scenarios (every case is unique—the list below is very broad, and for each person, the recommendation needs to be individualized):

1. Multiple prior early preterm births or second-trimester losses, especially if the cervix was dilated prior to birth without painful contractions. The more times this happens to someone, the more likely it is to be a cervical problem.

2. A prior preterm birth or second-trimester loss and a short cervix on ultrasound in this pregnancy (usually defined as less than 2.5 centimeters in length). The combination of a poor history and a current short cervix makes it more likely that there is a cervical problem.

3. A dilated cervix prior to 24 weeks without evidence of labor or infection.

If it is not clear if the cervix is weak, serial ultrasounds of the cervical length in pregnancy may help: you can plan to place a cerclage if the cervix shortens early in pregnancy (usually prior to 24 weeks) and not place a cerclage if it does not shorten.

There are other scenarios that are more controversial, like a short cervix on ultrasound without a history of preterm birth. For most women in this situation, a cerclage does not appear to be helpful, but there might be a subset who would benefit, like those with a very short cervix, or a cervix that is getting progressively shorter despite other treatments (like vaginal progesterone), or those with prior cervical surgery (LEEP or cone biopsy) or a uterine anomaly. If and when a cerclage is beneficial in twin pregnancies is also an area of controversy.

As this discussion makes clear, this decision is often extremely complicated and specific. It's one where you might well want a second opinion, from someone like a maternal-fetal medicine specialist.

The good news—in this chapter overall—is that usually we see things go better in a second pregnancy after a preterm birth. Typically, the second pregnancy does deliver later, or have a better outcome. This can either be directly related to our monitoring and interventions or simply because the first preterm birth was due to a nonrecurring cause. Either way, there is room to be optimistic and hopeful.

Bottom Line

- Recurrence risk for preterm birth is greater if the prior birth was more preterm.
- If the cause of preterm birth was cervical insufficiency (aka cervical incompetence), cerclage can lower the risk of recurrence.
- Progesterone supplements have mixed evidence and are worth discussing with your doctor but may not be universally prescribed.
- Plan for additional screening and ultrasounds if a previous pregnancy ended in preterm birth.

CHAPTER 11

Cesarean Section (and VBAC)

DEFINITION: Cesarean section: birth through abdominal surgery and hysterotomy (incision through the uterus)

OVERALL PREVALENCE: 35 percent in the US

RECURRENCE RISK GROUP: High (more than 50 percent)

An opening note on terms for this chapter: VBAC refers to vaginal birth after cesarean. Technically, you cannot choose to have a VBAC, because that would imply definite success. What you can choose is a TOLAC, a trial of labor after cesarean. If successful, this would lead to a VBAC.

This chapter is a bit different from many of the others. A cesarean section isn't properly a pregnancy complication; it's a safe and effective mode of delivery. A huge share of women in the US—as many as a third or more—deliver by C-section, and the rates of complications for both mothers and their babies are very low.

Based on randomized trials, outcomes for babies are not statistically different by birth mode.[1] For mothers, the short-term recovery from a C-section is slower (it's major surgery) but long-term recovery is similar. In fact, there are some long-term issues (pelvic organ prolapse, urinary incontinence) that are more common for vaginal births.[2] The most significant concern with a C-section is in risks in later pregnancies (more on this below).

If you had a C-section with a first pregnancy, it is likely that the default option in later pregnancies will be a repeat C-section (rather than a trial of labor with the hope of a vaginal birth). This default has changed some over time. In the first half of the twentieth century, the common adage was "Once a cesarean, always a cesarean." Beginning in the 1970s, this became less widely accepted, and vaginal birth after cesarean (VBAC) became more frequent.

Then, in the mid-1990s, a study published in the *New England Journal of Medicine* suggested that a repeat cesarean was a safer method of delivery.[3] After that point, the use of trial of labor after cesarean (TOLAC) declined (overall rates of cesarean section also increased over the years following). In the 2010s, there has been pushback against this, with more providers being open to considering a VBAC. And so, the pendulum is shifting, at least slightly, back in that direction.

Despite the recent shifts, this history, and the mid-1990s trial, mean that a repeat cesarean is still likely to be the default option offered.

For many women, this is a welcome option. As one woman told me:

• • •

My emergency c section was due to being stuck at 7 cms dilation and not due to harm to the baby. My actual c section was a pleasant experience and recovery was fast. I'm pregnant with my second and going to go for an elective c section. One, because my OB suggested that the reason for the first c section could manifest again in the second. Second, with a toddler home, planning the birth will take some of the stress out.

. . .

For others, though, this option is less preferable and they very much want to try for a VBAC.

Sometimes, this is because their recovery from an emergency C-section was traumatic. In some cases, women have labored for many hours only to find that the baby did not descend through the pelvis. The recovery from this—both emotional and physical—can be hard. You've done almost all of the work of vaginal birth *plus* major surgery.

The good news here is that for most people a second planned C-section is a much better experience. This shows up in my interviews with women about their birth experiences, but it also shows up in survey data.[4] In one study, women were asked about their satisfaction with their birth experience.[5] Out of a total of 10 (maximum satisfaction), spontaneous vaginal birth got an 8.86, versus 7.86 for elective cesarean. However, emergency cesarean delivery received only a 6.71. This is echoed in other data.[6]

Despite this, for a good share of women, attempting a VBAC is very important to them. As one woman told me:

. . .

I was very disappointed in myself about the C-section (even needing therapy to process it). I'm currently pregnant with my second and am strongly pursuing a VBAC—working with a birth center with high VBAC success rates and plan to hire a doula. I've been consumed with thoughts of the second birth experience, and I'm pretty worried about what my emotional state will be if VBAC isn't successful.

· · ·

Remember: a C-section is not a personal failure. In the end, this is really about preferences. And these preferences will naturally play a crucial role in what type of birth you pursue. But data is also a key input—there are risks and benefits to both options.

The ideal study here would be a randomized trial where a large number of women with one prior cesarean are randomly assigned to have a repeat cesarean, versus a trial of labor. Such a study would allow us to carefully calculate success rates, predictors of success, risks, and complications. This type of study is difficult to accomplish for a number of reasons. One issue is that many women (and their doctors) might not be amenable to having the decision taken out of their hands. Nearly all randomized trial evidence on pregnancy and birth choices relies on "encouragement designs"—people are encouraged but not required to adhere to one treatment or another—but these designs rely on at least some people changing their behavior due to the encouragement. In this case, a randomized trial would likely run into an issue where a lot of people did not adhere to their assigned group. This would make it hard to learn anything.

The best evidence we have comes from a 2013 Cochrane Review that found only one randomized trial that studied infant and maternal outcomes.[7] It had twenty-two women in it. The researchers did not find significant differences, but there is little to nothing to learn from that.

In lieu of having this kind of perfect data, we can piece together answers to our key data questions from various sources. Although these will not be perfect, they'll point us toward the important questions for this decision.

DATA QUESTION 1:
PROBABILITY OF SUCCESS

Most people do not attempt a VBAC (about 14 percent of women with a prior cesarean have a successful VBAC; based on average success rates this suggests about 18 percent of people try).[8] This makes it very difficult to get an unbiased sense of the probability of success. The issue is that the people who *do* attempt labor are likely to be those with a greater chance of success (doctors will be more likely to encourage or at least condone a trial of labor, for example, if they think it's more likely to be successful). This means, however, that the success rate for actual trials of labor will be, on average, higher than it would for the whole population.

Amplifying this issue is the fact that most of the data we have on success rates comes from academic medical centers. These hospitals may not be reflective of all care locations; the resources at a large academic medical center—easy and fast access to emergency care, for example—may make it easier to plan a trial of labor than it would be at a small community hospital.

With these caveats, the largest study of trial-of-labor success rates is based on almost 12,000 women studied at 19 academic medical centers.[9] Within this sample of women, 74 percent of them had a successful VBAC. There is, however, a lot of predictable variation in success rates by cohort.

Older age, higher prepregnancy weight, and small stature all lower success rates by a small amount. Much more important are obstetrical factors—namely, the reason for the prior cesarean. Success is much less likely (about half as likely, in the data) if the prior C-section was a result of a stalled labor (as opposed to, say, a planned C-section for a breech delivery). This probably reflects the fact that having a C-section for a stalled labor is informative about your physical ability to have a vaginal birth.

Conversely, success is much more likely (two to three times) if you had a vaginal birth before the C-section, and much, much more likely (perhaps six times as high) if you had a prior VBAC. This all makes sense—if the reason you had a cesarean was related to "the baby not fitting well" (that's not a real thing, but it's easier to conceptualize, and it includes reasons like a stalled labor or someone pushing for a long time and not delivering vaginally), it would stand to reason that the second time around, that issue might come up again. However, if it was due to a twin pregnancy or a placental issue or some other reason, it would stand to reason that the next time around, the likelihood of a vaginal delivery wouldn't be much less than for anyone having their first baby. Also, for someone who has delivered a baby vaginally before (whether before or after the cesarean), it also stands to reason that they should be able to do it again.

Returning to the analysis of the 12,000 women: The authors of the paper are interested in how much of the variation in the VBAC success rates they can account for by using the data they see. Their answer is that about 75 percent of the variation is explained. So, while it's not perfect, it has a lot of predictive power. This model is also translatable into a calculator.[10]

The calculator generates a predicted probability of success. For example, if you are 35 years old, 5'6", and 150 pounds, with no prior vaginal birth history, no arrest of labor, and no hypertension, your probability of success is calculated as 73.2 percent. That same person with a prior VBAC has a predicted success of 94.7 percent. But if the prior labor was arrested, the success rate drops to 60 percent.

The calculator may be helpful for discussions, although it's important not to put too much weight on individual numbers, which come with a lot of error. The most important takeaways from this data is that VBAC success rates can be high, and that the circumstances of the prior birth are among the most important factors.

DATA QUESTION 2: RISKS OF VBAC

The most significant risk associated with VBAC is uterine rupture. This is pretty much what it sounds like: the layers of the uterus rupture. Essentially, what happens is that the prior scar on the uterus is unable to withstand the forces of labor (contractions, maternal pushing), and it separates while the baby is still inside. It's rare, regardless of the mode of delivery, but it's extremely serious.

The risk of a uterine rupture with a trial of labor is estimated to be in the range of 0.5 to 1 percent. This risk appears to be slightly increased if labor is induced.[11] The fatality rate from uterine rupture is around 1 percent for the mother[12] and around 5 to 10 percent for the baby.

In the event of a uterine rupture, access to immediate emergency care is crucial. This may be a factor in considering a VBAC, depending on what type of hospital you plan to deliver at. If a serious complication happens while on a labor floor under the care of your doctor, the likelihood of a serious injury to you or the baby is approximately 10 percent. If it happens at home, on the way to the hospital, or at a facility unable to perform a cesarean quickly, the risk of a serious injury is much higher.

DATA QUESTION 3: RISKS OF A REPEAT C-SECTION

One downside to a repeat C-section is slower immediate recovery time. There's more on that in the fourth point.

With any cesarean, there are the risks of surgery itself. These include bleeding requiring blood transfusion, damage to other organs (intestines, bladder), and a hysterectomy (removal of the uterus). Fortunately, for a repeat cesarean, these risks are low, approximately 1 percent. It is important to note that the risks might be slightly *higher* if the cesarean is done on someone in labor, as opposed to someone coming for a scheduled cesarean. So when considering the risk of a cesarean, it is also important to consider that the risk of VBAC needs to also include the chance of a failed VBAC leading to a cesarean, which may have slightly more risk than a scheduled cesarean.

Perhaps the most significant consideration here is the risk that repeat C-sections may pose for later pregnancies. In general, the more cesareans, the higher the risk. Meaning: there are more risks for later pregnancies if you've had two cesareans than if you've had one, more for three than for two, and so on. The good news is that if you have a good surgeon for your C-section, the risks are still not extremely high.

The largest risks relate to the placenta, and, of these, placenta accreta (where the placenta is abnormally adherent to the uterus and is not delivered after the baby) is the most important concern. When someone has placenta accreta they cannot have a "simple" cesarean because when it is time for the placenta to come out, it doesn't detach fully, leading to massive hemorrhage and potentially even death. The treatment is usually (not always) a hysterectomy, and even in the best of hands, the recovery from a cesarean hysterectomy for placenta accreta can be long and difficult.

Overall, the risk of a placenta accreta increases with each cesarean. In addition, this risk is further elevated if you also develop placenta previa (where the placenta is located in the lower part of the uterus, covering the cervix). The baseline risk of placenta previa is about the same in each pregnancy (around 3 to 5 percent), but the risk of having placenta accreta goes up dramatically if you've had prior cesarean deliveries. For example, the table below shows the risk of having placenta accreta for patients with and without placenta previa, based on the number of prior cesareans:[13]

Cesarean Number	Approximate Risk of Placenta Accreta If You Do Not Have Placenta Previa	Approximate Risk of Placenta Accreta If You Have Placenta Previa
First	< 1%	3%
Second	< 1%	11%
Third	< 1%	40%
Fourth or higher	2%	> 60%

We can see evidence of the risk elevation in a 2018 meta-analysis that combined studies including almost 30 million births.[14] The authors compare long-term outcomes for women who had C-sections versus those who had a vaginal birth. In particular on the placental issues, they find a 75 percent increase in risk of placenta previa, and a 38 percent increase in the placental abruption risk. Most elevated is the risk of placenta accreta, which is three times as high in women who have had a C-section.

Given all of this, one of the key considerations in this choice is likely to be whether you plan on having more children. If yes, the benefit of avoiding a second cesarean is higher, as it will help you avoid your third or fourth. If you plan on only two children, the stakes aren't as high for the second birth (at least medically).

DATA QUESTION 4:
DIFFERENCES IN RECOVERY

The recovery from a C-section is, on average, longer and more painful than a vaginal birth. This is true for almost mechanical reasons—it's major abdominal surgery. Vaginal birth, to be clear, can also be quite traumatic and take a long time to heal from. But on average, there is a big difference. And there is certainly a difference in the "best case" scenario.

If you've already had one C-section, you probably have a sense of the recovery process. What may be important to keep in mind, though, is that the recovery from a planned and emergency C-section also differs. The physical (and in many cases mental) trauma of going through, say, eighteen hours of labor and then having an emergency C-section is very different from planning surgery in a predictable way.

This data point may be useful to keep in mind in combination with the predictors of success. A trial of labor that leads to an emergency C-section would be expected—based on these results—to yield lower satisfaction.

STRUCTURED DATA SUMMARY

In a sense, the trade-offs are straightforward to articulate.

A repeat C-section is predictable. It carries substantial recovery time, though is likely less traumatic than if your first was an emergency. There are elevated risks in later pregnancies.

A trial of labor is less predictable. There is a variable chance of success, based on your characteristics. A successful VBAC means, on average, an easier recovery and less risk to later pregnancies. An unsuccessful VBAC carries a small risk of serious complications and a larger risk of need for an emergency C-section.

This data summary may be helpful, but it doesn't give you the answer.

MEDICAL PERSPECTIVE

When thinking about decisions that should be made by you versus made by your doctor, VBAC is one of the decisions that really needs to be made by the patient, assuming it is a reasonable and safe option. In the majority of cases, from a medical perspective, neither a VBAC nor a scheduled cesarean is known to be definitively better. Each has possible benefits and risks, and, though the exact risks are different, the magnitude of the risk on both sides is about 1 percent. So when I am counseling someone about VBAC versus a repeat cesarean, unless there is a clear reason why VBAC is unsafe for them, I usually try very hard to let them decide which way to go. In this conversation, I will go over the individual-specific risks, the likelihood of success, and what each option looks like logistically. I then give the patient the choice (I am happy to help them with this choice if they want, of course).

I'm going to walk through that discussion here, to give you a framework to bring to your own conversations.

1. Is VBAC a safe option for me?

This is the first question that should be asked, because the answer is not always yes. The 1 percent risk of uterine rupture I quoted assumes that your first cesarean was done in the most common manner, a *low-transverse* uterine incision. Essentially, this means the incision on the uterus was made horizontally (left to right or right to left) in the lowest portion of your uterus. This type of incision tends to heal very well and has a low risk of rupturing in a future labor (approximately 1 percent). However, sometimes the incision on the uterus needs to be done vertically (top to bottom; sometimes called a *classical* cesarean), and if the incision reaches the middle or upper portion of the uterus, the risk of uterine rupture with a future labor is closer to 5 to 10 percent, which is considered too high a risk. Fortunately, almost all cesareans nowadays are done with a low-transverse incision on the uterus.

For this reason, many doctors want to see the operative report from your prior cesarean before answering this question. If you cannot get a copy of the report, it may be a deal-breaker for some doctors or hospitals (since they cannot formally document that you had a low-transverse cesarean). You certainly want to ask about this in advance if getting a copy of the operative report is infeasible. It is important to note that the scar on your abdomen does *not* indicate the type of scar on your uterus. Meaning, even though the scar on your abdomen is transverse and low, the scar on the uterus can be anywhere and in any direction. There is no reliable way to determine the details of the scar on your uterus without reading the operative report.

2. Is VBAC an option for me logistically?

You might be a terrific candidate to try a VBAC, but if you are seeing a doctor who doesn't do them, or delivers at a hospital that doesn't allow them, you need to either have a scheduled cesarean or go elsewhere. The earlier you know this, the better. There is no point in trying to argue your way out of this—it's not a good solution for them or for you. If your doctor isn't able to provide it and it's something you want, you may need to consider switching providers or hospitals (if that is possible).

It is also important to get a sense early on of how supportive of VBAC your doctor (and hospital) is. Even if they "allow" VBAC, if you are the only one in the building who wants you to have a VBAC, you are less likely to succeed. The trick is finding out this information. The simplest way might be asking an open-ended question like, "What is your general opinion on VBAC?" and see how the doctor responds. If they say, "I love them! I'm so happy when we can help someone achieve one," that is a lot more encouraging than "They're fine, I suppose, but in my experience, they are rarely successful and they're probably not worth the risk. But if you want one, I guess I'm okay with it."

This isn't a precise science, but most people will show you their cards if you ask them. As for the hospital, I recommend asking your doctor directly something like, "I am pleased you are supportive of VBAC. Is the hospital you deliver at also supportive? Will the nurses and staff try to support me as well?" If the doctor says that they themselves are very supportive of VBAC but the hospital is not, that's a tough call. You might want to see if there is another option, or at least have an open conversation with your doctor about how they might navigate that difference in attitude between themselves and the hospital.

3. What are my risks with either choice, and what's the likelihood of success?

Here is where the data from above comes in.

There are risks to a VBAC. Assuming you had a low-transverse cesarean, the risk of uterine rupture is approximately 1 percent. It is somewhat lower (0.5 percent) if you had a successful vaginal delivery prior, and it is somewhat higher (1 to 2 percent) if you had two prior cesarean deliveries, or if labor needs to be induced for this birth. The other risk is that a failed VBAC will lead to an emergency cesarean.

There are also risks to having a repeat cesarean. These include the risks of complications from surgery (about 1 percent) but also risks to future pregnancies. As noted, the weight of this consideration is very dependent on your future fertility plans. There are some instances when the risks of a cesarean might be higher (if you had other prior surgeries, for example). This is something your doctor will review with you.

Finally, there is the likelihood of success. The calculator Emily mentioned is somewhat useful, and between that and a conversation with your doctor, you should be able to find out if you have a lower

(50 percent or less), reasonable (approximately 75 percent), or high (greater than 90 percent) chance of success. The two biggest factors are whether you had a vaginal birth before (this is good) and whether your prior cesarean was for a reason related to a stalled/prolonged labor (not good).

I encourage people to consider these risks and likelihood of success together when making the decision. For example, you might view a 1 to 2 percent risk of uterine rupture much differently depending on the chance of a successful VBAC. It might be worth the risk to you if your chance of a vaginal delivery was 90 percent, but it might not be worth it if the chance was closer to 20 percent.

4. What do I want?

This is an important question that, amazingly, often gets overlooked. Not everyone wants a VBAC—it scares them, they don't like the uncertainty, they really don't want another long labor followed by a cesarean, or whatever reason makes sense to you. It is perfectly reasonable to *want* a repeat cesarean. It is *your* birth!

Decision Time

The goal of this discussion is to make a plan with your doctor for what you *intend* to do. It will generally fall into three choices:

1. I plan to try for a VBAC.
2. I plan to try for a VBAC, but only if I go into labor spontaneously by a certain gestational age (i.e., I want a VBAC, but if I need to be induced for some reason, I'd prefer the cesarean).
3. I plan to have a cesarean.

Once that initial decision is made, be open to moving from one category to another. For example, you may be in group 1 but then learn that your baby is estimated to be ten pounds at birth, and the last baby who didn't come out after you pushed for four hours was only seven pounds. Now you might want to move to group 3. Or perhaps you started in group 3, but you show up in labor a week before your scheduled cesarean and you are eight centimeters dilated, whereas for the last baby you had a cesarean because you never dilated past two centimeters. Now you might want to move to group 1. Or you started in group 1 but then find out you need to be induced in two weeks for mild preeclampsia and it is likely going to be a long induction, and now your risk of uterine rupture is slightly higher with the induction, so you move to group 2.

The main point is that the initial decision does not need to be considered the word of God. Circumstances change—your decision about a VBAC can change, too.

Sometimes it is important to take a step back from this decision and remember that in the big picture of the life and health of your child, whether you have a VBAC is probably not high up on the list of decisions you will make. Sure, take the time to research it and think about it, and make an informed choice that works best for you and your family, but keep it in perspective.

I say this with great humility, as I have never been in your exact shoes, but I have been around the block a few times as an obstetrician and a father of four (cesarean of twins, a VBAC for our third [forceps were needed, too!], then another VBAC for number four), and I can say with certainty that I rarely meet someone who thinks that much about their mode of delivery ten years after the fact, unless something went horribly wrong. So take it seriously, but always try to remember:

if the birth results in a healthy mom and a healthy baby, it is a big win, no matter how it happens.

Bottom Line

- Your probability of a successful VBAC depends on a number of factors. The most important is why you had a C-section previously; if it was for stalled labor, the chance of a successful VBAC is smaller than if it was for another reason (like a breech baby).
- The primary risk to a repeat C-section is a higher chance of placental complications in later pregnancies.
- The primary risk to a trial of labor is uterine rupture or (more likely but much less serious) the need for an emergency C-section.
- Make a plan with your doctor or midwife for your intended mode of delivery.
- To do this, take into account your specific risks, likelihood of success, and your personal wishes. Make a plan for what you want, but be flexible.
- If circumstances change during pregnancy, your plan can change as well.

CHAPTER 12

Severe Maternal Morbidity

> DEFINITION: Severe maternal complications during pregnancy, birth, or immediate postpartum
>
> OVERALL PREVALENCE: Low; varies across conditions
>
> RECURRENCE RISK GROUP: Low (less than 5 percent) for most conditions

In popular discussion, episodes of severe maternal complications are sometimes called birth trauma. We have avoided that language here, both because it's not precise and because a wide variety of birth experiences can be traumatic, even when they are not life-threatening for the mother. However, there is no question that severe, life-threatening maternal complications surrounding birth are incredibly traumatic for nearly all who experience them. They can also be incredibly traumatic for partners and family. An experience that is intended to be joyous, if a bit intense, is rendered with a completely different cast.

For many people who have severe maternal complications, the

idea of another pregnancy is completely out of the question. For some, the complication may have left them unable to carry another pregnancy. For others, it may be possible to do so but too risky or too frightening to consider. They may choose to grow their family in other ways. For yet another group, future fertility may remain on the table.

Regardless of the path, emotional consequences here are often significant. Women with severe maternal morbidity can have PTSD, and therapy can be a crucial part of managing care in a later pregnancy. For many of the women I talked to, even contemplating another pregnancy is either challenging or out of the question.

• • •

I have always wanted more than one child, as has my husband. However, after that delivery my husband absolutely wants no more children and I am extremely hesitant to try for more. The cardiology team strongly recommends we never get pregnant again. We are absolutely dumbfounded by this entire experience and currently trying to trudge through the trauma that we continue to experience daily.

• • •

More than anything, we want another so that the one we have can have a sibling. But the risk/benefit ratio is highly skewed to the risk and there seems to be no good reason to move forward with another. The complications of that delivery 100 percent will influence our final decision. It was a horrifying ordeal for us both, one that we never want to relive and something I am not willing to risk—at this time—for the sake of my precious, perfectly healthy and happy baby and his father.

• • •

After a fairly easy pregnancy, I had a traumatic birth in which I got sepsis, went into DIC [disseminated intravascular coagulation, which causes abnormal blood clotting] following an emergency C-section, and had significant complications from various interventions. I was delayed in meeting my daughter, had a long recovery, struggled with PPA/PTSD [postpartum anxiety/post-traumatic stress disorder], and struggled with breastfeeding. I so very much want another child, but the birth and postpartum period with my first was so challenging and painful that I don't know if I can do it again. I understand that in all likelihood a second experience would be different, but I now know what is possible, and that is very intimidating in terms of planning for a second child.

• • •

If you are in these types of situations, and you are considering another child, the experience of pregnancy management is likely to be very different. The rest of this chapter talks through a number of the most frequent causes of severe maternal morbidity. There is so much variation in this area that our goal here will be to give a big picture overview, with the understanding that your circumstances are likely to be very specific. For example, my hope is that if you had a postpartum hemorrhage, you will come out of this chapter with a better understanding of what this condition is and how it is treated. This is a bridge to your provider conversation, where the exact details of what happened are relevant.

These issues are medically complex, and their treatments are as well. In the following sections I'll give a brief overview and statistics on recurrence; Nate will dive into the medical details and treatment.

POSTPARTUM HEMORRHAGE

Postpartum hemorrhage (PPH) refers to a loss of a significant amount of blood during and after birth. This is by far the most common source of maternal complications, and it varies in severity. The current definition used in the US is: cumulative loss of more than 1,000 milliliters of blood (average blood loss is closer to 250 milliliters for a vaginal delivery and 600 milliliters for a cesarean) *or* bleeding along with signs of low blood volume (weakness, fatigue, dizziness). In severe cases, a blood transfusion may be required. Globally, postpartum hemorrhage is one of the top five causes of maternal mortality.

Postpartum hemorrhage is estimated to affect between 1 and 2 percent of births, but this depends on the definition and on how blood loss is measured (it is harder than you might think to quantify blood loss at the time of a delivery).[1]

Recurrence and Prevention

Prior PPH is a significant risk factor for later development. In one large study from Sweden, 15 percent of women who had PPH had a recurrence in a second pregnancy.[2] Overall, 5 percent of women had PPH overall, so if it happened before, the risk was three times as high. After two pregnancies with this complication, the risk was 26 percent.

The risk of recurrence depends on type. In some cases, excessive bleeding was a result of injury—either vaginal or cervical. If that's the case, the risk is less elevated in later pregnancies. In other cases, a recognized placental issue (like placenta previa) is responsible; this would increase the risk only if the issue occurred again. A common cause of PPH is uterine atony—a condition describing low uterine muscle tone—which would be more likely to recur in later pregnancies.

The primary approach to preventing PPH in a second pregnancy is more aggressive treatment with medications that cause the uterus to contract (i.e., oxytocin at higher doses after birth, or adding a second medication such as misoprostol or methergine). These are the same medications that would be used as a first-line treatment for uterine atony in any pregnancy, so it makes sense that they would work as a preventive measure as well for high-risk women.

STROKE

A stroke is when a portion of the brain is deprived of oxygen for a long enough period of time to cause damage to the brain tissue. The consequences of having a stroke depend on the size and location of the brain injury, and there is a wide range. Stroke is usually caused by decreased blood flow to an area of the brain, either because of narrowing of a blood vessel or sometimes bleeding from the vessel (so the blood doesn't get to the intended target).

Stroke is rare in women of child-bearing age, but women who are pregnant or recently pregnant are about three times as likely to have a stroke as women of a similar age who are not pregnant. The risk is the highest at the end of pregnancy and immediately postpartum.

Pregnancy-related strokes may be a consequence of preeclampsia (because blood vessels constrict), blood clots in the brain, bleeding in the brain, blood clots that form elsewhere in the body and migrate to the brain, or other causes. This isn't well understood.

As with any stroke, the prognosis varies tremendously based on the size of the stroke and its location in the brain. Recovery may be faster or slower, complete or incomplete.

Recurrence and Treatment

Similar to the case of PPH, the recurrence risk for stroke varies based on the cause.

For most causes of stroke, recurrence risk is low. For example, ischemic stroke (the most common pregnancy-associated stroke) has a recurrence rate during pregnancy similar to outside of pregnancy (about 1 percent).[3] Having had a stroke in a previous pregnancy is therefore not thought to be a contraindication to a later pregnancy.

There are some less common causes of pregnancy-associated stroke. For example, a condition called an arteriovenous malformation (AVM) in the brain is an uncommon but possible cause of stroke. If this is the cause, the risk of recurrence is much higher. As with much of this book, the more information you can get on your condition, the more effective later counseling can be.

In some cases, women who had a stroke in a prior pregnancy will be prescribed aspirin or another blood thinner. This depends, again, on the cause. For example, if the stroke was associated with preeclampsia, aspirin is clearly indicated.

BLOOD CLOTS (THROMBOSIS)

Pregnant women are generally at increased risk for blood clots. The two most common clotting issues are deep vein thrombosis (DVT), which typically appears as clots forming in the lower leg or thigh, and pulmonary embolism (PE), which appears as clots in the lungs. PE is usually secondary to DVT, meaning there was first a DVT, then the clot broke off from the vein in the leg, then it traveled through the bloodstream to the lungs, where it became wedged.

These risks of DVT and PE are higher in pregnancy for two reasons. First, there is more pooling of the blood in the lower extremities due to the physical changes of pregnancy. Second, blood clotting factors tend to increase during pregnancy. There are evolutionary reasons for this: clotting factors are valuable in lowering bleeding during birth. Because of this elevated risk, you'll see caution against long-haul flights during pregnancy, which themselves can be a risk for blood clots.

Still, although risks in pregnancy are elevated, they are overall low. In a retrospective study of about 70,000 women in the UK, the incidence of DVT was 0.7 per 1,000 deliveries, and the incidence of PE was 0.15 per 1,000 deliveries.[4] These figures are small relative even to other serious complications, like postpartum hemorrhage.

Recurrence and Prevention

There is an elevated risk of recurrence after an initial thrombosis. In one study, which followed 189 women who had thrombosis in an earlier pregnancy, 17 of them (8.9 percent) had either DVT or PE in the following pregnancy.[5] On one hand, that means that 90 percent of them did not have this. But given the low overall risk, it is hugely elevated relative to baseline.

Treatment during a subsequent pregnancy will typically involve blood thinners, though precisely which ones will depend on the circumstances in the first pregnancy. Beyond that, you'll likely be intensively monitored for possible recurrence.

PERIPARTUM CARDIOMYOPATHY

Peripartum cardiomyopathy is a (very rare) cause of heart failure that occurs later in pregnancy or during the early postpartum period. It is not specifically associated with the time of birth. Women with cardiomyopathy will have the same symptoms as anyone with heart failure: severe shortness of breath, extreme weakness, fluid in their lungs, chest pain.

There is a large range of estimated incidence, depending on geography. In the US, estimated risks range from 1 in 1,000 to 1 in 4,000, but, again, this is not based on compelling evidence, likely due to inconsistent reporting of this condition as "peripartum" when it first presents weeks or months after delivery. What we can say is that it is quite rare. There are large racial and ethnic differences in incidence, with Black women having a higher risk of the condition and higher risks of serious versions.

Recurrence and Treatment

This condition is extremely serious, and is associated with high rates of mortality and morbidity. Women who have heart failure during pregnancy are more likely to have heart issues after pregnancy. The risk of recurrence is high, and generally those who have had this condition are recommended against getting pregnant again, unless it was a relatively mild presentation with complete recovery afterward.

SEPSIS

Sepsis is a complication of infection that can lead, in extreme cases, to organ failure and death. This can occur post-birth as a result of infection. It is rare. In one review of 44 million deliveries, sepsis occurred in 1 in an estimated 3,333 and severe sepsis in 1 in 10,800.[6] In the past decade, there has been increased focus on sepsis and sepsis prevention, and many hospitals now have sepsis alerts and sepsis protocols designed to recognize and treat infections early to prevent sepsis or the consequences of sepsis. As a result of this more intensive monitoring regimen, many more women giving birth are being given a diagnosis of sepsis or possible sepsis.

For women who do not otherwise have an immune deficiency, sepsis largely occurs randomly as a result of an infection. Infections can occur with any injury or surgery, including those associated with birth.

Recurrence and Prevention

Recurrence for most causes of sepsis is low. Having had a sporadic infection at one time doesn't dramatically increase your risk at another time. In these cases, no additional treatment would be necessary in a later pregnancy.

An exception to this is that (rarely) sepsis can be a complication of kidney infections (pyelonephritis). This would have a high chance of recurrence in later pregnancies, and frequent monitoring (with urine cultures) and possible treatment with prophylactic antibiotics may be necessary.

MEDICAL PERSPECTIVE

As a general rule, most women who have a severe complication at or after birth, such as the ones Emily listed, are otherwise healthy. As such, the risk of recurrence is low. That said, there are some women with a severe complication who do have an underlying predisposition or condition in which the recurrence risk would be higher and the management of a future pregnancy and delivery potentially much different. Because it may not be obvious which category you fall within, anyone with a severe complication at delivery really should have a consultation with an OB-GYN or MFM as soon after the pregnancy as possible to review what happened, undergo any needed tests, and plan for a future pregnancy.

I will use PPH as an example, as it is one of the more common causes of severe maternal morbidity.

The proximate cause of most PPH (about 80 percent) is "uterine atony"—when the uterus does not contract properly after birth.

Normally when we bleed (like when someone accidentally cuts their finger), the way the body stops the bleeding is by sending a bunch of clotting factors, or proteins, to the cut. We can think of them as plugging the hole. If the cut is too big or too deep, sutures are needed to close that gap and stop the bleeding.

Bleeding after a delivery is very different. Most of the bleeding after delivery comes from the blood vessels that are in the uterus traveling toward the placenta. When the baby is delivered and then the placenta detaches from the uterus, there are large blood vessels exposed that bleed at an extremely rapid rate—as fast as 1,000 milliliters per *minute*. This could not be stopped in time by clotting factors. The uterus stops bleeding by contracting tightly around those vessels (like stepping on a garden hose). If this doesn't happen, bleeding can continue, the amount of which will depend mostly on how uncontracted the uterus is and for how long.

Other causes of PPH include retained placenta (a portion does not come out), large vaginal or cervical tears, and, rarely, a deficiency in clotting factors (they aren't the main way we stop bleeding after birth, but they are still much needed).

Anything that would reduce the ability of the uterus to contract constitutes a risk factor for uterine atony and therefore PPH. This includes a long labor, infection, an overdistended uterus (from twins or high amniotic fluid volume), and a history of PPH in a prior pregnancy (see below). Other risk factors include larger babies, forceps and vacuum deliveries, a long labor, and preeclampsia. One big risk factor that gets overlooked is cesarean delivery. Since the average blood loss is higher with a cesarean, there is also a higher chance of losing a large amount of blood.

There are certain placental problems that are directly causal to PPH, so they technically wouldn't be "risk factors." For example, placenta previa and placental abruption are both causes of heavy bleeding in pregnancy, during delivery, and potentially after delivery as well.

Treatment for PPH depends on the severity and the particular cause; however, it is an emergency and will be treated as such. Usually, PPH is treated with some combination of uterine massage, a variety of medications, a balloon placed in the uterus temporarily to tamponade the bleeding, and occasionally embolization of the uterine arteries (done by an interventional radiologist). In rare instances when none of the other treatments work, an emergency hysterectomy is needed to save the life of the woman. In these cases, more pregnancies will not be possible. Fortunately, in the vast majority of cases, the bleeding can be stopped without removing the uterus, and future pregnancies may then be possible.

When I meet someone with a prior PPH, we spend most of the time reviewing her history and medical records to try to determine the cause. This will help me estimate the likelihood of recurrence, as well as potential interventions to reduce the risk, or at least treat it earlier, reducing the total blood loss.

Similarly, with other pregnancy complications, the most important part of this workup tends to be a thorough history, a review of whatever medical records and test results are available, a detailed history of any prior pregnancies, along with a full medical, surgical, gynecological, and family history. At times, I will do a physical exam or an ultrasound of the uterus. Typically, this provides enough information to determine if any additional tests are needed to rule out any underlying conditions. Sometimes I will refer patients to a different specialist (such as a cardiologist, hematologist, or neurologist).

Once the story is clear and all the testing is complete, we usually meet again, or at least speak on the phone, to review the results and plan for the next pregnancy. Often we determine there is nothing to do and that the risk of it happening again is very low. Sometimes I will recommend increased monitoring or certain treatments in the next pregnancy or delivery. Sometimes my patients will also need to follow up with one of the other specialists mentioned above.

As ever, planning is key. For some people, looking ahead is the best way to get everything set before the next pregnancy. For others who are undecided if they want to try again, having a sense of what the pregnancy would look like and what the risks might be enables them to make that choice. Contrary to what many people assume, it is actually pretty unusual for us to conclude that it is too dangerous to have another pregnancy. For example, in my group practice of ten maternal-fetal medicine specialists doing several hundred preconception consultations a year, it probably happens once or twice a year.

Once a plan is in place and you are pregnant again, working through the fear of the complication recurring is a crucial next step. Since most of the complications we are talking about happened at or right after delivery, the fear often peaks at delivery, and so reassurance during delivery and postpartum can be a necessary support. Some of this is already built into the medical plan (like additional treatments at delivery or more frequent monitoring after delivery), and some of it is simply addressing whatever anxiety might be present, which is going to be different for everyone.

Ultimately, if you had a severe complication and had the appropriate evaluation and workup, you will know well in advance what the risks of another pregnancy might be. And since they often turn out to be low, or manageable with good care and follow-up, a healthy pregnancy and delivery is happily the most common outcome the next time around.

Bottom Line

- In most cases, the risk of recurrence of these conditions is low.
- Consult with an OB-GYN or MFM between pregnancies to go over what happened and map out a plan for the next pregnancy.
- This might require a consultation or continued follow-up with other medical specialists.
- Develop a plan for mental health support during pregnancy.

CHAPTER 13

~~~~~~~~~~~~~~~

Stillbirth

DEFINITION: A fetal demise after 20 weeks of pregnancy

OVERALL PREVALENCE: Estimated 0.6 percent of
pregnancies

RECURRENCE RISK GROUP: Low (estimated 2.5 percent)

I n the United States, *stillbirth* is defined as the birth of a baby with no
sign of life after 20 weeks of gestation. (Globally, the definition sometimes starts only later, at 28 weeks, but we'll use the US definition here.)
Before 20 weeks, fetal loss is documented as a miscarriage. Between 20
and 27 weeks of gestation it's an "early stillbirth," between 28 and 36
weeks a "late stillbirth," and at or after 37 weeks a "term stillbirth."

When a stillbirth occurs, the pregnant woman may know of the
fetal demise in utero before delivery or it may be discovered at the
time of birth. With the use of fetal monitoring in labor, it is very unusual nowadays to have a stillbirth not identified prior to birth.

Stillbirth is more common than many people think. I do not say
this to scare you; it is still a low risk. But like many things in pregnancy

(miscarriage, birth trauma, complications), the fact that we do not discuss it means that, if it does happen, people can feel much more alone than necessary.

There are about 23,000 stillbirths a year in the US; that's about 1 per 160 deliveries.[1] This is about 40 times lower than the risk of first-trimester miscarriage, but it's higher than the risk of Down syndrome and other chromosomal conditions. About half of these stillbirths are early—before 27 weeks—and half are after.

A stillbirth is among the most traumatic experiences that a woman can have during pregnancy. In many cases, it is completely unexpected. In the words of one woman: *My first daughter (first pregnancy) was stillborn at 35+6 in January 2020. I noticed she hadn't moved since the previous night, we went in, and she had died.*

In other cases, there is a precipitating medical event—*We lost our first, Jack, in 2019 at 36 weeks to a catastrophic placental abruption with an unknown cause.*

However it happens, the moment of learning of fetal demise is a devastating one for nearly all families (and providers). If it occurs in utero, the fetus will ultimately need to be delivered (with the process depending on the fetal age). In many cases, a fetus will be delivered vaginally, with induced labor. Depending on your wishes, it should be possible to hold the baby after birth, to say goodbye. You can also take photos and have footprints or other keepsakes made.

As with any pregnancy loss—but likely more so here—there is an enormous grieving process to go through after a stillbirth. There are resources at the end of this chapter to connect with others who have gone through similar experiences.

If and when you do find yourself ready to try again, we must ask whether it is likely to happen again.

WHAT THE DATA SAYS:
RECURRENCE AND PREVENTION

To begin to talk about risk of recurrence, it is helpful to start by talking about the causes of stillbirth. To be clear: in many cases, the cause
of a stillbirth is unknown. It is not always possible to do further testing or an autopsy—many families do not want this—and sometimes
the cause is simply unclear, even with that information.

Having said that, there are a few known causes, many of which
overlap with those for miscarriage and premature birth.

- *Genetic/anatomic/metabolic abnormalities.* Fifteen to 20 percent
  of stillbirths have notable abnormalities or major malforma-
  tions, or can be identified as having a chromosomal abnormality. Chromosomal abnormalities are a cause of a very large
  share of first-trimester miscarriages; in some cases, these issues are compatible with further development but not live
  birth. As genetic testing has become more advanced, more
  cases of stillbirth are being attributed to genetic causes, and
  the actual percentage due to genetic abnormalities is likely to
  be higher than 20 percent. Similarly, when autopsies are performed on stillborn babies, a genetic, anatomic, or metabolic
  abnormality is identified 20 to 50 percent of the time.
- *Infections.* An estimated 10 to 20 percent of stillbirths are caused
  by maternal infection. Listeria, *E. coli*, cytomegalovirus (CMV),
  parvovirus, and Zika are among the causes.
- *Placental abruption.* Five to 10 percent of cases are a result of
  placental abruption, a condition in which the placenta detaches

completely or partially from the uterus. This is sometimes a result of physical trauma (for example, a car accident) but is usually spontaneous.

- *Umbilical cord event.* An estimated 10 percent of stillbirths are a result of an umbilical cord event (a knot in the cord, for example). A note here is that umbilical cord issues arise with some frequency (20 percent of healthy babies have a cord around the neck, for example) and almost always cause no significant issues whatsoever, so it is sometimes difficult to know whether a cord issue is really at fault or just a coincidence.

- *Fetal growth restriction.* Growth-restricted fetuses (those that are growing more slowly than expected) are at higher risk of stillbirth. This is not itself a cause, and in some cases it's a result of one of the causes cited here (for example, genetic abnormalities). But fetal growth restriction can also be a sign of placental dysfunction, and it may be this dysfunction that is the cause in these cases.

- *Thrombophilia.* This is when there is an increased likelihood of blood clotting in the mother's own circulation, which is hypothesized to increase the risk of stillbirth by causing clots along the placenta. The clots reduce blood flow through the placenta, decreasing its function and reducing nutrients and oxygen to the fetus, leading to stillbirth. The data supporting a link between most *inherited* forms of thrombophilia (like Factor V Leiden, prothrombin gene mutation, and protein C or S deficiency) and stillbirth are tenuous, and it remains unclear if these conditions are a cause of stillbirth and if treating them with blood thinners like heparin and low-molecular-weight heparin are helpful in the next pregnancy. For those with *acquired* thrombophilia—namely, antiphospholipid antibody syndrome (an autoimmune disorder)—there is more evidence suggesting it is associated with stillbirth, especially if the stillbirth is preceded by fetal growth restriction or preeclampsia. Therefore, it is usually recommended that patients with a prior stillbirth be tested for antiphospholipid antibody syndrome and if the test is positive, take blood thinners in the next pregnancy.

- *Placental insufficiency.* This is when the placenta function declines either slowly (more common) or rapidly (less common) to the point that it is no longer able to provide the nutrients and oxygen needed for the baby to thrive, eventually leading to fetal death. This manifests as fetal growth restriction, low amniotic fluid, and sometimes placental abruption or preeclampsia. Placental insufficiency is more common as pregnancy progresses past 39 or 40 weeks, which explains why post-term pregnancy (after 42 weeks) is also a risk factor for stillbirth. It is also more common with several maternal factors such as older age, infertility treatments, higher body mass index, certain medical conditions, and multiple pregnancies, and it at least partially explains why these are all risk factors for stillbirth.

Even aggregating all these together, at least half of stillbirths are for unknown reasons. This can be devastating for families looking for answers.

Recurrence

Women who have had one stillbirth are at elevated risk for a second stillbirth, relative to those who had a live birth with a first pregnancy. A 2015 meta-analysis calculates that the risk of stillbirth in a second pregnancy is three to five times as high for those who had a stillbirth with a first pregnancy.[2]

There are two very important pieces of context for these data. The first is that although the relative risk is significantly elevated, the absolute risk is small. In the meta-analysis, among those who had a stillbirth in the first pregnancy, 2.5 percent had a stillbirth in the second pregnancy. This is substantially elevated relative to the overall risk in the population, but it still means that 97.5 percent of those women had a live birth in a second pregnancy. So the recurrence risk is elevated, but as a probability it is low.

The second important context is that the risk of recurrence varies tremendously depending on the cause (if it is known). A stillbirth due to a placental abruption after a car accident does not translate to a recurrence risk. Similarly, an infection isn't likely to recur. On the other hand, stillbirth that is a result of fetal growth restriction may suggest a more elevated risk.

For this second reason, if there are opportunities to learn about the cause of a first stillbirth, it is a good idea to take advantage of them.

Prevention

As a baseline, if you had a stillbirth, you will have more monitoring in a later pregnancy. This is true whether or not the cause is known.

Some of the issues that raise the risk of stillbirth—like fetal growth restriction—are more likely to be identified with more extensive prenatal monitoring. In addition, it is common and natural for expecting parents to be more anxious about a pregnancy following a stillbirth. More frequent prenatal check-ins can be crucial for partially alleviating this anxiety.

A second point is that if the cause of a stillbirth was identified, there may be treatments that address that particular cause.

First, induction at term. There is evidence to support a policy of routinely inducing labor for all women by 41 weeks. A randomized trial in Sweden published in 2019 found that stillbirth rates were significantly increased when doctors waited until 42 weeks to induce.[3] So induction of labor by 41 weeks is highly recommended.

For those with a prior stillbirth, it is very likely that you'll be offered an induction at 39 weeks or earlier. In the past, there were concerns that routine inductions might lead to an increased risk of C-section (in general, not necessarily for women at risk of stillbirth). However, in 2018 a large randomized trial in the US (called the ARRIVE trial) showed that induction at 39 weeks of pregnancy had similar outcomes (similar risk of C-section, similar outcomes for moms and babies) to waiting for labor to start on its own.[4] The result has been a move toward offering inductions to everyone at 39 weeks, regardless of their risks. For mothers with a prior stillbirth, this is even more likely to be suggested.

Beyond this, even though induction of labor prior to 39 weeks is not routinely recommended due to the small increased risk of neonatal complications, for women with a prior stillbirth, delivery at 37 or 38 weeks is sometimes offered or recommended either because of the risk of recurrence or because of extreme maternal anxiety, especially if the previous stillbirth was prior to 39 weeks.

A second, commonly cited intervention with the potential to lower stillbirth risk is counting kicks. There are many ways to do this, but the most codified one is the "count to ten" method: periodically (say, once a day), you see whether there are at least ten movements you can perceive over the course of two hours. The idea is to stop when you get to ten, which takes an average of twenty minutes. Another method is to count for thirty minutes—if there are at least three movements in thirty minutes, that is reassuring.

The logic behind this approach is sensible. Decreased fetal movement is frequently detected prior to a stillbirth, and this kind of systematic approach is easy to explain and implement. It seems logical that it might catch some cases and allow for intervention.

The empirical data on kick counting is not as compelling as one might think based on the logic.[5] The largest trial of this approach, the AFFIRM study, included 400,000 women.[6] The authors did not find a significant impact: the control group had a stillbirth rate of 4.4 per 1,000, versus 4.06 in the intervention group. This is about a 7 percent decrease, but not large enough given the sample size to show significance. Other studies have similar results. The primary downside to this intervention is possible added stress and unnecessary doctor visits.

So kick counting continues to be a common intervention, but this data suggests that its impacts, if they exist, are likely to be small in magnitude.

A final approach worth mentioning given the links between stillbirth and the placenta is the possibility of placental measurement. A lower placental volume has been linked in the data to lower birth weight and fetuses that are small for their gestational age.[7] This suggests that placental measurement could be a marker for increased risk. I say "suggests" because, of course, it could be that some third factor is responsible for both a small fetus and a small placenta. But identifying this has the possibility—in theory—of marking people for increased follow-up.

Placental volume has generally been hard to measure in utero (the study mentioned above uses an MRI, which is not standard in pregnancy). However, recent research has suggested that an estimate of placental volume can be derived from straightforward ultrasound measurements.[8]

This approach has yet to be tested in large-scale trials, and routine measurement of placental volume isn't recommended. It shows potential, but nothing close to certainty. Also, for someone with a prior stillbirth, it is unclear if placental volume would be a useful tool, because the only "treatment" for someone with an abnormal placental volume is to do serial measurements of fetal growth, which is likely going to be recommended for someone with a prior stillbirth regardless of placental volume.

MEDICAL PERSPECTIVE

Unfortunately, I see a lot of women with a prior stillbirth. It is definitely more common than people think, and the pain that it causes cannot be overstated. This is true at the time of the loss, of course, but it is also true during the next pregnancy. For this reason, when I see someone with a prior stillbirth, we probably spend about 50 percent of the time talking about the possible cause of the loss and the testing and treatments we can try, and the other 50 percent of the time talking about mental health. I am not a formal mental health care provider (psychiatrist, psychologist), but I have found that talking about it openly is both comforting and helpful to patients and their family going through another pregnancy. So this section will also focus on both the medical and the psychological care of pregnancies after a stillbirth.

Medical

Ideally, conversations with your provider begin between the loss and the next pregnancy. Trying to ascertain the cause of a stillbirth can take some time; there are some tests that are best (or only) done between pregnancies, and occasionally there are treatments that need to start prior to or early on in pregnancy. For example, if the cause was a genetic abnormality in the fetus, it would be very important to know prior to the next pregnancy if it was a mutation carried by the parents. If so, you could choose to conceive through IVF and test the embryos for this mutation and only implant embryos without the mutation. For all of these reasons, if you had a prior stillbirth and are considering another pregnancy, I would recommend scheduling a preconception consultation with your OB-GYN or midwife, or a maternal-fetal medicine specialist.

Getting data from the prior pregnancy is extremely helpful. This includes doctor notes, laboratory results, ultrasound reports (or even images), genetic screening and testing results, and the results of a pathological examination of the placenta or an autopsy of the newborn, if one was done. These data can identify a cause, or a likely cause, about 50 percent of the time. The other 50 percent are attributed to either a cord event or an unknown cause. For these reasons, for someone going through a stillbirth, I always strongly recommend a thorough workup at the time. Most of this is noninvasive, such as blood tests for the mother and pathological examination of the placenta, including genetic testing. Autopsy is understandably a difficult decision for parents, especially those planning a burial for their child. I do recommend autopsy to increase the chances of finding a cause of the stillbirth, but I also totally understand those who simply are not able to agree to this.

During the consultation, I try to get a thorough review of what happened in the previous pregnancy. This includes hearing the full story from the patient and her partner (or any other family member or friend who was involved), and I often ask a lot of specific questions about timing of events, symptoms, bleeding, and exposures. I always recognize that bringing up the story of the loss is likely going to be painful, but it is definitely important. It is both understandable, and common, that the recounting of the story is very emotional, tearful, and sometimes needs to be done piece by piece. Also for this reason, it might be helpful for you to write down in advance all the details of the loss you remember. This can be done at your own pace based on how difficult it is for you, but when it is complete you can either send it to your doctor in advance of the meeting or bring it with you.

When I am meeting with a patient, if the cause of the stillbirth was unknown and the testing was not done at the time of the stillbirth, I recommend testing for antiphospholipid antibody syndrome and sometimes inherited thrombophilias as well (case by case). If she hasn't been screened already, I test for diabetes, hypertension, and thyroid disease. Similarly, if she has not been screened, I will recommend expanded carrier screening for her and potentially her partner. I will sometimes recommend an assessment of the uterine cavity with a saline infusion sonohysterogram or MRI.

In the next pregnancy, I usually recommend supplementation with a prenatal vitamin, calcium, and low-dose aspirin. If she has antiphospholipid antibody syndrome, I will also recommend heparin or low-molecular-weight heparin. If we chose to test for inherited thrombophilias and she has one, I might recommend heparin or low-molecular-weight heparin as well. If she has medical conditions, we will try to get them optimized prior to her next pregnancy.

Also, I typically recommend frequent office visits and ultrasounds, both to have objective evidence that this pregnancy is progressing well, which consequently reduces anxiety by giving frequent reinforcement that the baby is doing well, and ample time for you to ask questions and just talk. Most women with a prior stillbirth require visits every few weeks early in pregnancy and, as they get closer to the time of delivery, much more frequent visits. My baseline schedule for women with a prior stillbirth is visits every two weeks until 32 weeks and then weekly or twice weekly until delivery. We are happy to accommodate women who want more or fewer visits. The weekly or twice-weekly visits from 32 weeks include a formal assessment of fetal health, either as a biophysical profile (ultrasound) or nonstress test (prolonged tracing of the fetal heart rate pattern). This might start as early as 28 weeks, especially if the previous loss was earlier.

I do not routinely have women with a prior stillbirth do formal kick counting for two reasons. First, we are already doing a formal assessment of fetal health. Second, I don't need to—as soon as they feel anything is off, they are usually calling our office asking to come in anyway.

Timing the delivery depends on many factors. Assuming all the testing is normal, and with the above strategy, the actual likelihood of a recurrent stillbirth is very low, probably in the 1 percent range. That said, 1 percent is not zero, and regardless of the risk of recurrent stillbirth, as pregnancy progresses the anxiety often increases significantly and can become quite painful. Many women with a prior stillbirth who are now 37 weeks with a healthy pregnancy just want that healthy baby delivered. If there is a small chance the baby needs to go to the NICU, they would rather take that chance than go home with the extreme fear that they will wake up the next morning with another stillbirth. For this reason, I typically recommend delivery anytime after 37 weeks, based on her exact history and her own anxiety level. We review the risks and benefits of all options, and anyone who wants to deliver at 37 weeks, that's usually fine with me. In my experience, that is what most people choose the first pregnancy after a stillbirth. If not 37 weeks, then usually 38 or 39 weeks.

Psychological

As you may have already learned, I'm a pretty peppy-positive guy, but I don't want to sugarcoat this: the pregnancy after a stillbirth is awful.

I don't write this to scare you, nor to dissuade you from trying again. As I've noted, with close monitoring the chance it will happen again is very low. However, I find that many women and families simply are not prepared for the emotional tornado a second pregnancy can fuel. At the time of the loss itself, there is tremendous grief and despair, and with a lot of time that usually improves. But of course, it's never gone, and it often returns with the next pregnancy. At the same time, there is the expected anxiety and fear that it is going to happen again, and during the pregnancy this gets worse with time, not better. On top of that is a component of post-traumatic stress from entering another pregnancy. Then, the guilt. Guilt over the previous pregnancy (Was it my fault?), guilt over joy you might feel in this pregnancy (How can I

be happy when I lost a baby?), and guilt over grief you feel (How can I
be sad when I have this healthy baby inside me?). Of course, *all* the
guilt is unwarranted, but that's how guilt goes—we feel it anyway. Putting the grief, anxiety, fear, trauma, and guilt together makes this very
hard.

But it is doable. Pregnancy is temporary, and with a lot of support,
you can get through it. The following are a few suggestions I give to
women and couples with a prior stillbirth. Not every suggestion is right
for everyone, but these are some things I have learned over the years
working with many women to help them go through a pregnancy after
a stillbirth. They are not in any particular order.

1. *Radical acceptance.* Sometimes knowing and accepting that you
   are going to be extremely anxious takes some of the sting off the
   anxiety. I have found that there is the anxiety itself and then
   there is the meta-anxiety, or the dismay over being so anxious. I
   try to reassure women that it is totally *normal* to be so anxious
   in this pregnancy and to accept it, rather than fight it. Or em-
   brace the fact that you will be a wreck. It's both allowed and
   expected.

2. *Support.* You will need help from someone or everyone: family,
   friends, support groups, books, podcasts, anything. Everyone is
   different in what they need and from whom, so try to find who
   is helpful to you and lean on them (with their permission). Also
   find the people who are the opposite for you, and avoid them as
   much as possible.

3. *Expect some people, even people who love you, to disappoint you.*
   Most people have no idea what you went through with the loss
   and what you are going through with the next pregnancy, so even

though they care about you and want to be helpful, they may not know how. They may also say some pretty painful things, simply out of ignorance. For example, you are likely to hear "Things happen for a reason" or "This baby will be a comfort for your loss" and other comments that may be hurtful. Try to ignore these comments. They are intended to help, even though they don't.

4. *You may need formal mental health care by a professional.* Even if you never needed to see a psychologist, psychiatrist, or other mental health provider after your loss, or you did but no longer do, you may need to follow up with one during this pregnancy. Again, everyone is different, but don't assume that since you aren't currently seeing someone, you won't need to during the pregnancy.

5. *Make sure you are seeing a doctor or midwife who knows you are different from the "typical" patient.* It should be pretty obvious the first time you meet them if they have any clue what you are going through. If they do, you will probably feel a lot more supported during the pregnancy than if they don't.

6. *You are allowed to be selfish.* There are times in our lives when we are in a position to give and help, and other times when we are in a position of needing others to help us. The same person can be very giving one day (or year) and very needy the next. If you find yourself being the latter because of the pregnancy, just be open with your inner circle that this is one of those times you may not be as available for them, and that it is not because you don't love them but because you are going through something very difficult and you don't have the capacity right now to be that person. But one day you will be.

One of the most rewarding aspects of what we do is working with families who have gone through a stillbirth and partnering with you in the next pregnancy. We are continuously humbled by your strength and resolve. We are here for you.

Bottom Line

- With most causes of stillbirth, the risk of recurrence is low.
- Labor induction at 39 weeks is recommended.
- Kick counting may give some reassurance.
- Based on the cause of the stillbirth, you might require additional tests or treatments prior to or during pregnancy.
- Regardless of the cause of the stillbirth, you should have frequent visits to formally assess the baby and to give reassurance. The exact frequency will depend on how many weeks pregnant you are and your own personal level of anxiety.
- Do not underestimate how difficult the next pregnancy will be from a mental health perspective. Assemble a strong support system for yourself based on your own needs and preferences.

Post-Birth
Complications

CHAPTER 14

Recovery Complications

DEFINITION: Sustained physical injury or
symptom post-birth

OVERALL PREVALENCE: Varies

RECURRENCE RISK GROUP: Intermediate (10 to 50 percent),
but typically less severe

When I was in graduate school, long before I had children, a close friend and his wife had their first child. We visited them a couple of weeks later, and I have a very vivid memory of his wife opening the door, my asking "How are you?," and her replying—somewhat cheerfully—that she was fine other than a muscle tear all the way from her vaginal opening to her anus. I cannot remember what I said, but I hope it was nice.

The physical recovery from childbirth can be daunting, no matter how delivery goes. A very large share of women who have a vaginal birth have some degree of vaginal tearing. A cesarean section is major surgery. With either mode of delivery, you are likely to have moderate to heavy bleeding initially, and some bleeding through perhaps six weeks postpartum.

Healing takes time, no matter how a birth goes, and it will take more time if complications arise. However, we barely even talk about recovery from a "typical" childbirth experience. Recovery from more severe injury is even less discussed. This can leave people feeling alone, or like they are overreacting to a normal experience. In the words of one woman:

• • •

I only realized with time how different my recovery was from others' due to having fourth-degree tearing. Sitting was hard for the first six to eight weeks, making breastfeeding and going anywhere by car hard. Having nothing to compare it to and just having to get through it, that's what I did.

• • •

This, in turn, can decrease the chance that people get help to heal, or advice about how to manage another birth. In this chapter, I'll talk through some of the most common complications that arise post-childbirth, with an eye toward the question of later pregnancies as well as treatment.

It is important to note that in a number of cases, these conditions are something that may need attention and treatment even if you *do not* choose to have another pregnancy. Prolapse, for example, is a complication of a vaginal birth in which some internal organs can fall into the vagina. This has significant impacts on women, and requires treatment, even if there are no additional pregnancies. The same can be said of pelvic pain, which may interfere with daily activities or make sex painful. Urinary incontinence is in this category, too.

In all of these cases, there are treatments that can help. This chapter, then, may be useful for those who had a complicated recovery path, regardless of future fertility plans.

VAGINAL TEARING

In broad strokes, severe vaginal tearing is less likely in subsequent pregnancies. Nonetheless, before talking about recurrence, it may be useful to review details of vaginal tearing in general.

Vaginal tearing is very common during vaginal birth. The most common tearing occurs in the perineum, the muscle between the vagina and the anus. Vaginal tearing is described by degree.

- *First-degree tear*: small injury to the most superficial layer of tissue in the vagina and perineum
- *Second-degree tear*: slightly larger and deeper than first-degree, extending into the vaginal and perineal muscles
- *Third-degree tear*: a tear that extends from the vagina and involves the anal sphincter (the doughnut-shaped muscle around your anus), involving both the skin and muscle tissue
- *Fourth-degree tear*: a tear that extends from the vagina, entirely through the anal sphincter, and then into the rectum

It is also possible to have small tears in the labia. These are usually the depth of first-degree tears.

In first births, about 90 percent of women have some kind of vaginal tear. However, only a small share of these are the more severe third and fourth degree—one large study in the UK puts this figure at 7 percent in first births—with only 0.3 percent having fourth-degree tears.[1]

Third- and fourth-degree tears are the ones that have more potential for long-term issues given the involvement of the anal sphincter, which is the muscle needed to hold in your gas and stool. They are sometimes collectively referred to as OASIS, for obstetrical anal sphincter injuries.

A first delivery itself is a risk factor for third- and fourth-degree tears, as are larger babies. Operative delivery (with forceps and vacuum) is another.

The relationship between severe tearing and episiotomy is complicated. There is significant data showing that a policy of routine episiotomy (where more or less everyone gets one) results in more vaginal trauma than a restrictive use policy.[2] Routine use of episiotomy is therefore not recommended. However, there are cases in which the use of episiotomy may be appropriate.

Recurrence and Prevention

In general, tearing is less likely and less severe in later pregnancies. In the UK data above, third- or fourth-degree tears occur in only 2.7 percent of later births.

Having had a severe tear before, the risk of recurrence is higher. But it is still low. In one study, recurrence was 2 percent among those with prior severe tears, versus 0.3 percent among those without.[3] Another study put it at 10 percent among those with prior severe tearing.[4]

Perhaps the largest analysis of this, run in Australia, actually found *no* increased risk of severe tearing if you had a serious tear before.[5] It did find that women were slightly less likely to have a later pregnancy after a first with vaginal trauma.

There are not many strongly evidence-based approaches to preventing tearing, either initially or in recurrence. One that does have some support is perineal massage during labor. In a meta-analysis of nine randomized trials, the authors found a 50 percent reduction in the risk of severe trauma with vaginal massage during labor.[6] (To be clear, this isn't a spa massage. It's someone stretching your vagina with lubricated, gloved fingers.) Although it is common to add warm compresses to this, the evidence doesn't seem to suggest they further help.[7]

For women with a prior fourth-degree tear, many will choose an elective cesarean in the next pregnancy. The recovery from a fourth-degree tear can be extremely difficult, and reconstructive surgery may be required. In some cases, the elevated risks of recurrence, given the serious consequences, make a cesarean the right choice. As one woman told me:

. . .

It was important to both my husband and me to give our son a sibling, so I never questioned a second pregnancy, just knew that I would have more control over delivery. I had my daughter in September 2022 via C-section and could not be more pleased with my recovery. We do not plan to have any future children, but should we change our minds, I will 150,000 percent have a repeat C-section!

. . .

VAGINAL PROLAPSE/PELVIC ORGAN PROLAPSE

Vaginal prolapse or pelvic organ prolapse refers to a condition in which the pelvic floor muscles weaken to the point where some of your organs may collapse into the vagina. This can include the upper muscles of the vagina, the uterus, the bladder, or the rectum. This may or may not be painful, and you may or may not notice it. In cases of prolapse, you may be able to feel one of these organs in your vagina, or possibly protruding out of your vagina. This sounds scary, and it can be uncomfortable, but it isn't dangerous.

While up to 50 percent of women have some prolapse, it is largely asymptomatic. Symptomatic prolapse occurs 3 to 6 percent of the time.[8]

Prolapse is not a birth injury in the same way that vaginal tearing is. However, it is associated with childbirth, as the experience of pregnancy, and vaginal birth, raises the risk.

Recurrence and Prevention

The risk of prolapse goes up with each pregnancy, and particularly with each vaginal delivery. For women with no children, estimates suggest 0.6 percent of them have pelvic organ prolapse; after one birth, this increases to 2.5 percent. After two or three, up to almost 4 percent.[9] If you have a form of prolapse after a first pregnancy, it is extremely likely to continue through a second pregnancy, and may possibly get worse.

Prolapse is treatable—in less severe cases, with physical therapy; in more severe cases, with surgery. It is not a reason to avoid another pregnancy, but it is a good idea to discuss with your doctor to see if it makes sense to treat this with more physical therapy before pregnancy or plan to treat it after.

Surgical treatments are not usually performed until you are done having children, as they would either prevent another birth or likely need to be repeated again after the next birth.

WOUND COMPLICATIONS

Any wound can become infected. Post-birth wound infections are more common with cesarean sections than vaginal births, because the wound is typically larger. But both can happen. Most infections require antibiotics, along with frequent cleaning and packing with sterile gauze. This can be messy, painful, and scary, but it almost always heals well.

Infection is more common when a wound is closed with staples rather than sutures.[10] It is also more common if the cesarean section followed a long labor or was an emergency.

Recurrence and Prevention

There is a risk of recurrence for infection, but it is difficult to put in exact numbers. One preventive approach is prophylactic antibiotics, especially for a repeat cesarean section. This has been shown to lower the risk of recurrent infection.

MEDICAL PERSPECTIVE

For pelvic floor difficulties like prolapse and incontinence, I am a strong advocate for early assessment for anyone with symptoms that are not resolving and I will refer them to a pelvic floor physical therapist, a pelvic floor surgeon, or both. I also believe in early treatment, or even preventive treatment, for these issues. The only exception to this proactive approach is that it sometimes makes sense to postpone any surgery (if needed) until after you are done having children.

Of the recovery issues discussed in this chapter, the one that we discuss most in the context of later pregnancies is vaginal tearing.

As Emily noted, vaginal tearing (aka laceration) is more the rule than the exception for first births. For most women, the tear is first or second degree, heals relatively quickly, and, aside from one to three weeks of soreness, usually has no lasting effects. For these women, the risk of tearing in the next pregnancy tends to be lower, and the recovery the next time around also tends to be easier and faster.

For women with OASIS (a third- or fourth-degree tear), the recovery might be similar to a first- or second-degree tear, but often it is more painful and takes longer to heal. This is normal for these more advanced tears. A small percentage of women with OASIS have persistent issues, such as pain, as well as weakness of the anal sphincter, causing a decreased ability to hold in your gas or stool, and these issues are clearly very significant. For this reason, anyone with OASIS needs close follow-up after birth, and if there are any issues, even slight, they should be addressed quickly. Some women will benefit from pelvic floor physical therapy, others simply need more time, and a small percentage will need surgical procedures to strengthen or reconstruct the anal sphincter (these are *not* the types of operations that wait until you are done having children).

For women with a history of a fourth-degree laceration, which has the highest risk of complications and probably the highest risk of recurrence, I always discuss cesarean as an option for the next birth. It is the most reliable way to avoid another OASIS. I also think that if you had a fourth-degree laceration last time and your doctor or midwife has not offered a cesarean for the next birth, you should ask them to discuss this option, especially if you think you might prefer a cesarean. In my experience, most women with a prior fourth-degree laceration, when given both options, choose to deliver the next baby by cesarean. But some women prefer another vaginal delivery. These decisions would likely differ based on your own experience with your first OASIS, how many children you plan on having, and your own thoughts about cesareans.

A word about episiotomies. This is something where the pendulum really has swung back and forth and probably deserves to be somewhere in the middle. Episiotomies used to be the norm for vaginal deliveries. The thought at the time was that a surgical incision was easier to repair than a natural, more jagged tear, and that it would heal better as well, with less pain and complications. Also, there used to be less routine use of fetal monitoring, so the thought was that anything that delivered the baby more quickly was better for the baby (episiotomies can speed up delivery by several minutes). Subsequent to this, there were several large studies comparing routine use of episiotomy with more restrictive use. These studies showed that routine use of episiotomy did *not* lead to improved outcomes for mother and baby. In fact, for the mother, routine episiotomy was associated with a *higher* rate of OASIS. Based on these studies, pretty much everyone in the US stopped doing routine episiotomies.

However, some people went so far as to say that episiotomies should *never* be done. Episiotomies were described as "barbaric" and "debilitating." In the studies that showed that routine use of episiotomy was not the best strategy, the other group with restricted episiotomy had an episiotomy about 20 percent of the time, not 0 percent of the time. Since then, there have been a lot of guesses about what is the "best" rate of episiotomy, and they have ranged from 0 to 20 percent, most falling somewhere under 10 percent. But it is important to realize that nobody actually knows the ideal rate. Plus, any given person either gets one or doesn't—no single person has a 10 percent episiotomy. There are times when episiotomy is probably the best option for you. For example, if I see that there is going to be a lot of tearing upward toward the urethra, or in multiple places, it might make more sense to do a small episiotomy to have only one tear in a less painful location rather than multiple tears that may extend into very sensitive and painful locations. Or, if I am going to do a forceps delivery, I will often recommend an episiotomy and direct it *away* from the anal sphincter to reduce the risk of the tear extending into a third- or fourth-degree laceration. Basically, the ideal rate is definitely not 100 percent, but it's not 0 percent, either. Whether someone needs one is a judgment call, and the decision is hopefully being made by someone with clinical experience and good judgment.

I think the important thing here is not to establish the ideal rate but to make sure that you and your doctor or midwife are on the same page regarding episiotomy, and this is best discussed during your prenatal care as opposed to when you are already in labor. There are times when it is reasonable to do an episiotomy, and I would suggest asking your doctor or midwife how they decide when to do one. If the answer is "I do them 100 percent of the time," you should consider seeing someone else. Alternatively, if the answer is "I never do them," "I've never done one," or "They should never be done," I would also be wary. Ideally, your doctor or midwife will be able to talk with you about when they think it is reasonable to do an episiotomy and why. Based on that conversation, you are best able to gauge whether they are reasonable, thoughtful, and experienced, and whether their philosophy aligns with yours.

Bottom Line

- Vaginal tearing is a common recovery complication; the good news is that it is typically less severe with later pregnancies.
- After a very serious vaginal tear, you may consider a C-section to avoid recurrence.
- Prolapse and incontinence are common complications of vaginal birth that may get worse after multiple pregnancies. There are treatments that can help! Find a pelvic floor therapist if you're suffering from these complications.
- Postpartum pelvic floor issues like prolapse and incontinence that are not improving on their own should be evaluated and treated as early as possible.
- Episiotomies should no longer be done routinely, but they still do have a role in select deliveries.

CHAPTER 15

Postpartum Mental

Health Conditions

DEFINITION: Postpartum diagnosis of depression,
anxiety, or psychosis

OVERALL PREVALENCE: At least 10 to 15 percent of women

RECURRENCE RISK GROUP: High (more than 50 percent)

Postpartum depression and anxiety are extremely common. The onset can be shortly after birth or even months later. Many women discount later-onset depression, thinking postpartum depression happens only right after the baby arrives. This is not the case. It can also begin in pregnancy, in which case it is called peripartum depression or anxiety.

The prevalence of postpartum depression, even if we focus only on diagnosed cases, is high. An estimated 10 to 15 percent of women who give birth experience it.[1] The data suggests that about half of these women actually experience the onset of depression during pregnancy;

post-pregnancy, the diagnosis is most typical in the first four months after birth.

It is important to distinguish postpartum depression from postpartum mood changes, sometimes called baby blues. Postpartum depression is a defined mental health diagnosis that is by definition not part of the "normal" postpartum experience. It is different from occasional episodes of feeling overwhelmed or sad, which are *extremely* common (50 percent or more). The simplest way to differentiate them is that postpartum depression is when those feelings become persistent and affect your ability to function normally (sleep, eat, work, interact with others, care for your baby or other children, etc.). This distinction should be made by your doctor or midwife. You should report *any* of these symptoms, and they can help determine if you have postpartum depression.

There are some risk factors for postpartum depression. These fall into two categories: predisposition and situation. By far the biggest risk factor for postpartum depression is predisposition, or prior experience of depression. If you've had episodes of depression before, they are more likely to crop up again in the pregnancy or postpartum period.

The other risk factors are largely situational. Some of these factors are modifiable, and some are not. New parents who have less social support, who experience difficult life events around this time, or whose baby has medical or other problems are more likely to be depressed. And the baby itself can also play a role; people with babies who are poor sleepers are at greater risk for depression, almost certainly due to the fact that they, in turn, get less sleep.

The first identification of postpartum depression is often through a screening questionnaire—the most widely used is the Edinburgh

Postnatal Depression Scale. Many midwives and obstetricians give it at the six-week postpartum visit, although this doesn't always happen (which is a problem). Many pediatricians also screen parents for postpartum depression because they typically see the babies many times between birth and six weeks, so they usually have earlier and more frequent regular contact with the mother. An abnormal screen does not mean you have postpartum depression or anxiety (which is precisely why it is called a screening test and not a diagnostic test); it just means you should be evaluated formally for it, or followed closely to see whether your symptoms get better or not.

Much of the literature, and popular discourse, focuses on postpartum depression. But not all postpartum mental health issues take the form of depression. Postpartum anxiety is also common. Many of the symptoms are similar to postpartum depression, and, indeed, it is common to diagnose postpartum anxiety using the same screening tool. But women with postpartum anxiety also tend to find themselves fixated on terrible things that could happen to the baby, unable to sleep even if the opportunity is there, and engaging in obsessive-compulsive behaviors around infant safety or feeding or sleeping. This can be treated with therapy or, in more severe cases, with medication.

With anxiety, it can be hard to know where the line is between normal parental worry and obsessive worry. If anxiety is interfering with your ability to enjoy spending time with your baby, if it is occupying all your thoughts and preventing you from sleeping—that is over the line.

Less common but much more severe is postpartum psychosis. This affects an estimated 1 to 2 in 1,000 women and is much more likely to develop in women with a history of bipolar disorder.[2] Postpartum psychosis usually manifests in hallucinations, delusions, and manic episodes. The horrible stories you might have heard about women who harm their babies tend to be due to postpartum psychosis, not postpartum depression or anxiety. Self-harm, however, can occur with any of the diagnoses.

Postpartum mental health struggles can have enormous impacts on how families think about subsequent pregnancies. I heard from a lot of women and families about the impact this had on their decision making.

In some cases, women told me that the possibility of this happening again simply made it impossible to consider another pregnancy.

. . .

The influence of PPD [postpartum depression] was so strong on myself and my partner that it was the deciding influence on having a second child. Though two years postpartum, it is still incredibly hard thinking about that phase of parenthood. Basically, I just cannot imagine going through it again personally, but also the influence it would have on our firstborn. I had a very easy pregnancy and birth, so it almost feels trite and selfish for PPD to so strongly influence my decision, as I know many women have harder stories than mine. I know I will always be sad about not having another child, but I feel like we have to make decisions based on what's best for the family unit.

. . .

Other women focused on what they did differently the next time:

. . .

I started Zoloft six weeks prior to my due date in my second pregnancy and hired a night nurse in advance.

. . .

And still others expressed ambivalence and unanswered questions about whether the experience would change their future fertility path.

. . .

I have always wanted more than one child, and I still do. That said, the trauma of my birth and postpartum mania, insomnia, and severe postpartum depression for several months after my first child in some ways makes me dread going through the pregnancy, birth, and infant process again. I have learned a lot from the first time through and feel confident that things can and will be different a second time around, and will do everything in my power to make that so. But I've also learned that there is a lot that is just not in your control when it comes to birth and postpartum, and getting myself willingly involved in another round of birth and postpartum feels a little scary. All of that said, the joy my 16-month-old daughter brings me now, and the bond and connection we have, feels priceless. I wish I hadn't gone through such complex postpartum emotional issues, but I do know now that it was worth it for what was waiting on the other side.

. . .

Inherent in all of this is the concern about recurrence. I'll talk about the data in the following section. This is a clear case where there is both a pessimistic and optimistic spin. Having had postpartum mental health issues in an earlier pregnancy puts you at a much higher risk in a later pregnancy. However, being aware of the risks is a huge step toward getting better. Postpartum mental health issues often take a very long time to diagnose because they can be unexpected. If you know you are at risk, you can get help faster.

WHAT THE DATA SAYS: RECURRENCE AND TREATMENT

Recurrence

The most significant risk for postpartum mental health struggles is prior experience with them, either outside of or during a previous pregnancy.

This can be seen in a variety of studies. One large-scale example is a 2017 paper from Denmark.[3] The authors of this paper take a cohort of about 450,000 women and follow them over almost twenty years. Their metric of postpartum depression is contact with a hospital or a history of antidepressant medication, so they are looking at somewhat severe outcomes.

They find that among women who took antidepressant medications postpartum with a first pregnancy, about a third do so again. Among those who had psychiatric hospital contact after a first pregnancy, half of them do so again. These risks are about twenty-five times as high as they are for women who did not have these diagnoses.

These numbers likely understate the recurrence of depression of any severity, since not all postpartum depression would be treated. And given the enormously elevated risk for someone with prior depression, this falls into the "high" risk category: recurrence is more likely than not.

Treatment

Preventing depression may be challenging. But preventing it from having the most severe impacts should not be. Treatment is crucial. And, by extension, the key to treatment of depression is recognizing it. Evaluations of postpartum depression screening tools have shown as much as a 60 percent reduction in depression a few months later.[4] This isn't because the screening tool itself does anything! But once the issue is recognized, treatment can begin.

Treatment for postpartum depression proceeds in stages, beginning with therapy, exercise, and maybe improvement in sleep hygiene. For more serious depressive states, medication is prescribed. These can be used safely while breastfeeding.

In 2023, the FDA approved a new type of medication for treatment of postpartum depression specifically, called Zuranolone. This drug is taken for a short period—just fourteen days—and studies showed it provided fast improvements in depression, sometimes within just three days. This drug has not yet been evaluated for women who are breastfeeding.

If you have been through this before, you will know what works for you. The most important thing is to be on top of it. Get a copy of the depression screening, and do it regularly—don't wait for the doctor. Be prepared.

MEDICAL PERSPECTIVE

When I meet with anyone who has a history of postpartum depression or anxiety, or anyone with a mental health diagnosis like anxiety, depression, or bipolar disorder, we discuss the increased risk of depression and anxiety during the next pregnancy or postpartum. I usually tell them that there is good news and bad news. The bad news is that they have a high chance of getting postpartum depression or anxiety. The good news is that they are less likely to *suffer* from it. The majority of suffering that happens from postpartum depression and anxiety is during the time period between it starting and it being diagnosed. This can sometimes be many months. Not every woman knows when her symptoms are indicative of depression, and not everyone gets screened postpartum (unfortunately; everyone should be). Therefore, many women suffer for a very long time before getting the treatment they need.

The same is not true for someone with a history of postpartum depression or a chronic mental health condition. These people will immediately know when they don't feel right and will get the treatment they need much sooner. Therefore, they suffer less.

For this reason, I am typically very encouraging about another pregnancy. If you have a mental health provider you work with, continue to do so. Let them know you are pregnant or considering another pregnancy, and they will likely follow you closely in the next pregnancy and postpartum. If you are not currently seeing a mental health provider, I recommend connecting (or reconnecting) with one during pregnancy so you can have that relationship established and a plan in place should you have worsening symptoms at any time.

Some women even start (or restart) medication before birth or right after birth in the next pregnancy to avoid any recurrence. This decision obviously needs to be individualized based on your own history, experience with medication, and your and your mental health provider's attitude toward medication use.

Regardless of the specifics, as long as you are aware of your symptoms and have good mental health care, the likelihood is that the second pregnancy and postpartum period will overall be a better experience from a mental health perspective than the first one.

Bottom Line

- Recurrence of postpartum mood disorder is very likely.
- Effective screening and prompt treatment can greatly improve outcomes.

CHAPTER 16

~~~~~~~~

Breastfeeding Barriers

DEFINITION: Any condition that makes
breastfeeding challenging

OVERALL PREVALENCE: Varies based on condition

RECURRENCE RISK GROUP: Varies based on condition

Before I had my first child, Penelope, I had naively assumed that breastfeeding would just "work," or at least that I would quickly figure it out. I had not reckoned on a complicated set of interlaced problems. My milk took a long time to come in ("delayed lactogenesis"), and I had an overall low supply. Penelope only liked to nurse on one side, and actually didn't even like that too much. One of my breasts got much larger than the other and, honestly, they never really equalized.

There were many things that were more complicated about having my younger child, Finn (mostly, that I had the older child, too). But breastfeeding was one thing that was much, much easier. My milk came in faster, there was more of it, and, probably because of these factors, he was a happier nurser.

Even if it's working well, there are challenges to breastfeeding. Conditions like mastitis (a painful inflammation, and sometimes infection, of the breast tissue) can crop up at any time, and the sheer logistics of nursing, especially if you're working and pumping, are daunting.

One huge difference between breastfeeding a first child and a later child is that you've done it before. For some of the hard stuff, simply having been through it before can totally change the experience. It took me months with Penelope to figure out a good pumping schedule; by the time Finn came along, all I had to do was remember. Even with a condition like mastitis—which is just as bad the second time around—there is some peace in knowing the warning signs and how to treat it.

We should also say here that there is often a lot of pressure, from outside and possibly from yourself, to breastfeed because "breast is best." In my 2019 book *Cribsheet*, I wrote extensively about what the data really supports in terms of breastfeeding benefits. The short summary is that while there are some short-term benefits to the baby breastfeeding early in infancy—digestive health, lower risk of eczema—they are small. And the long-term benefits cited (including higher IQ and better long-term health) just do not seem to be supported in the best data.

Breastfeeding may absolutely be something that's important to you, that you want to do, that works for you and your family. This is a great reason to try to figure out a way over earlier barriers. But if it doesn't work for you, if the better choice for your family is formula, then this data may provide some helpful perspective.

The array of breastfeeding struggles is wide, and it may not be feasible to cover all of them here. What we can do is discuss the recurrence risk (and any treatment) for some of the more common struggles. It is also notable that we have, on the whole, quite limited data about issues in breastfeeding. What we have is better than nothing, but it's often not much.

WHAT THE DATA SAYS: RECURRENCE AND PREVENTION

Delayed Lactogenesis II

"Lactogenesis"—milk production—comes in two stages. Lactogenesis I occurs during pregnancy, when the breasts are preparing for milk production. In some women, small amounts of milk can be expressed as early as 16 weeks, and colostrum (the highly concentrated first kind of milk your body produces) starts to appear for most women at the end of pregnancy.

Lactogenesis II is the stage at which copious amounts of milk are produced. This occurs after birth, typically within two or three days. There is no formal numerical definition—it's not like this occurs as soon as you can pump some specific number of ounces—but generally women know when it happens.

Lactogenesis II is considered "delayed" if the onset is more than three days postpartum (after seventy-two hours). This is common. In one study of almost 2,500 women, 23 percent had delayed lactogenesis.[1] This delay can lead to a frustrating experience with early breastfeeding, causing some women to quit altogether.

Delayed lactogenesis is much less common in later births. In that study of 2,500 women, the condition occurred in 33 percent of first births and only 18 percent of later births. It is even lower for later births where there was breastfeeding experience with the first child.

Having said this, delayed lactogenesis in a first birth is likely to increase the risk with a later birth, simply because there are some underlying hormonal risk factors that are unlikely to have changed between pregnancies. Precise numbers on this are not available in the data, perhaps in large part because we do not do enough research on breastfeeding.

Prevention of this condition in a later birth may be possible in part by recognizing it. Earlier breast stimulation—more pumping after birth, for example—can increase milk speed and production.

Supply Issues: Low Supply, Oversupply, IGT

Your breast milk supply with an earlier birth is likely a good clue about the future. This is true for biological reasons—with similar stimulation, different breasts produce different amounts of milk. But either the first or the second time, it can seem like a Goldilocks situation: either too much or too little. Never just the right amount.

There are many factors that determine breast milk production, and the exact process by which some women produce more or less is not completely understood. Experimental approaches to trying to produce a lot of milk suggest that for most women, potential breast milk production is significantly higher than the needs of a single infant.[2] In other words, adequate supply is usually possible.

The most important modifiable determinant of breast milk supply is demand. Greater demand for milk—from your baby, from a breast pump—stimulates greater production. There are other factors that may matter—maternal stress during nursing, excessive weight loss—but for the most part, things like nutrition, fluid intake, and age and number of children do not seem to be influential.[3]

The recognition of the importance of the supply-demand feedback loop is a clue to thinking about issues of low supply and oversupply of breast milk. If your supply was low with a first birth, the solution may be more demand. This could involve adding pumping sessions early on, which will stimulate more milk production. If your supply was too high in earlier births, avoiding this type of extra pumping early on is a good idea.

There is one case in which this is unlikely to work, which is if you were diagnosed with insufficient glandular tissue, or IGT. This condition is rare—the medical literature is largely limited to case reports, so it's not even clear what the overall prevalence is—but it is caused by insufficient development of the breasts' milk-making tissue at some earlier stage. With this diagnosis, it may not be possible to produce enough milk even with great effort. If this diagnosis was made with an earlier child, it will carry over to a later one.

Latching Problems

Many people struggle with latching during early breastfeeding. The most common sign of this is significant nipple pain. While nipple soreness is experienced by a large share of breastfeeding women in the first week or two of life, continuing nipple pain beyond that is not expected and can interfere with the continuation of breastfeeding (in addition to just being painful and unpleasant).

Latching struggles can often be addressed with repositioning, and, if you worked through this with a first child, you're likely to be able to apply some of those lessons. The prevalence of nipple pain is lower—perhaps only half as much—among later births versus first births.[4] This suggests that there is substantial learning that takes place.

Ejection Reflex Issues

When a baby starts nursing, they suck for a few seconds and then the milk "lets down." There are two issues that are sometimes associated with this letdown.

First, for some women, the milk release is very aggressive. A lot of milk comes out—it can be almost shooting out. And this initial burst of milk can be overwhelming for a baby and cause choking, hiccupping, etc.

It's not well understood *why* this happens or how common it is.

If you struggled with this issue before, you are likely to struggle with it again. And the solutions are likely to be the same: pull the infant off the breast in the first phase of letdown, pump briefly before nursing, try to nurse lying down so gravity pulls in the opposite direction. Solving this problem is mostly about coming up with a solution that works for you and then implementing it.

A second issue: the letdown reflex is associated with a surge of hormones. For some women, this surge can leave them feeling sad, anxious, or panicked. This is sometimes referred to as dysphoric milk ejection reflex, or D-MER. The prevalence of this condition is not well understood. One study reported a prevalence of 9 percent, but it recruited from a sample of people in support groups oriented toward this condition.[5] That will dramatically overstate the prevalence.

Again, if you struggled with this before, it seems likely that the second time will be similar. Lack of data prevents us from saying *how* likely it is.

If you struggled with breastfeeding a first child, it makes sense to be proactive about it before a second child arrives. For this, the office visit you want is not with a specialist like Nate but with a lactation consultant. Your doctor is great, but except in unusual situations, they are not likely to have extensive training on the topic of breastfeeding.

The group with official training in breastfeeding support are lactation consultants. Among these, the ones with the most training are those who are certified as IBCLCs (international board certified lactation consultants). A variety of websites (for example, lactationnetwork .com) can help you find someone with this qualification.

An important caveat to this is that if you struggled with breastfeeding after a first birth, you might have had experiences with lactation consultants. And those experiences might not have been good ones. In some cases, the process of lactation consulting can seem more like advocacy than support. Women can be made to feel like breastfeeding struggles are their failure, or they can be pushed to nurse beyond what actually works for them and their family.

This is not an argument for not getting outside support! It's an argument for finding someone in this space who can help support the goals you have for yourself.

Before you visit any office, begin by thinking about what you want this time around. Here are some questions to start with:

- Do you want to breastfeed at all this time?
- What were the primary issues last time?
- What do you want to be different this time?
- How long do you hope to nurse for?

Once you've answered these questions honestly for yourself—especially the first one—you're in a much better position to talk with an expert and find one who aligns with your values.

The goal of the office visit during pregnancy should be to make a plan for what support you'll need, when you'll need it, and what the details of nursing will look like. If you had trouble with latching early on, how can you get support for that right away? If the issue was low supply, what steps are there in the plan to (perhaps) pump more in the first days?

In these discussions it is also worth considering the added complications that having another child present will bring. Even if nursing is more familiar, having another person to take care of (get off to school, etc.) can be a challenge.

In the end, breastfeeding a first child is a totally new experience. Breastfeeding a second child isn't. You have more time, and more knowledge, to figure out what works for you. Many things may be the same, but your preparation for them will not be.

Bottom Line

- Breastmilk tends to come in earlier on average with a second child.
- Other issues (low supply, overactive ejection reflex) often recur with a second child, but may be easier to manage given more experience.
- Evaluate your own desire to breastfeed again.
- Talk with a supportive lactation consultant before birth.

CHAPTER 17

Conclusion

I first contemplated writing this book because of conversations with people who had questions about what data would be helpful to have before embarking on their next pregnancy journey. Because of how I write, where my expertise is, and the focus of my work, this book is largely an answer to these questions. What does the data say? How can I use evidence to make the right decisions, and maybe to have a different outcome next time?

Those conversations are not why I wrote this book, though. The ultimate decision to write this, to devote a book to talking through the details of the hardest parts of pregnancy, came down to two conversations.

The first was with Kaleigh Summers, a psychotherapist who is herself a survivor of an episode of severe birth trauma. We talked about the idea of later pregnancies after severe complications. What she told me was that many people she's worked with come to the second pregnancy with an idea of redemption, that a different outcome this time will erase the prior experience. If everything goes well, that will be enough to allow someone to move on.

In her experience, that was rarely the case. A second pregnancy wasn't necessarily a rescue, and processing whatever loss, grief, or trauma was there in the first place was still necessary.

Although much of the focus in this book is on how to approach a second pregnancy, in nearly all cases the first part of this is looking carefully back at the first. Part of my hope is that in looking back, there will be a moment for some processing. For what Nate calls "radical acceptance."

The second conversation was a series of emails that began with an email asking for my advice, from a woman who was facing a possible second-trimester pregnancy loss after her cervix dilated too early. In our first emails there was fear, but also hope. But then she wrote a few days later to say that her son had been born, and it was too early for him to survive.

She and I emailed on and off after that, as she approached another pregnancy. I could feel the fear, and still also the hope. And then, one day, an email with the subject "Sharing News" and a picture of her with just-born son, sharing a middle name with his older brother. Echoing the first point, this didn't erase the memories or ease all the trauma, but the email and the pictures were just pure, unadulterated joy in that moment.

This is, ultimately, where I hope the readers of this book can come to. The recognition first that what happened was hard and needs to be processed, not just ignored. But also, the realization that there can be joy.

Acknowledgments

Books do not appear out of thin air, and this is no exception. I'm grateful to Suzanne Gluck for helping me see the way to writing this one, and the others. I will forever be in Ginny Smith's debt for her firm, but gentle, guidance and for scoping on this particular book on a tiny hotel notepad with me. Caroline Sydney played a second huge editorial role here; thank you, Caroline. The whole team at Penguin Press deserves thanks: Ann Godoff, Scott Moyers, Matt Boyd, Danielle Plafsky, Elisabeth Calamari, Aly D'Amato, and Meg Gerrity.

The team at ParentData also deserves thanks for all their help with this book, and with the ParentData universe: Alex Birch, Katie Salam, Sophie Taylor, Denisse Myrick, Jasmine Thomas, Tamar Avishai, and Nadia Schreiber.

The group in some ways most deserving of thanks is nameless—but it is you, the people who reached out with your questions and inspired this writing. Whether you're writing on Instagram, to the Q&A, to my email, you mattered for this book.

I am sorry I didn't write you back! I wish I could write back to everyone, to answer every question. Hopefully this book answers some of them. I'm so grateful to you for trusting me with your stories and your hopes and struggles and dreams. It is the privilege of my life to get to be there with you, in some small way, in the good and the bad moments. Special thanks to Kayleigh Summers for guiding me through the birth trauma discussion here.

Thanks to Nate for writing with me! It was great fun. I could not have asked for a better partner.

To my family: Dad, Steve, John, Rebecca, Andrea, James, Emily, Connor, Matthew, Maya, Marcus, Simone, Joyce, Arvin, Emily, Terence, Leila. Thank you for the support, and the love.

Mom, I miss you.

Jesse, Penelope & Finn: you three put up with a lot. I know how lucky I am to have you. I love you.

—Emily Oster

Thank you, Emily, for deciding one day to pivot and start writing about pregnancy, and for being so awesome at it. You are changing people's lives for the better, and as a doctor I really appreciate it. I also thank you for answering that very first email from a random, occasionally inappropriate, obstetrician and MFM in New York and then being so available to speak, meet for lunch, collaborate on several projects, and appear as a guest on my podcast so many times. I have learned so much from you about data, explaining data, and communicating with parents, and my patients and listeners continue to adore you. I have never written a book before, and I could not have asked for a better partner. You are a dream coauthor: pleasant, efficient, and smart. But, most importantly, you are one of the most gracious people I have ever met. Although you are clearly the famous one of us two, the Batman to my Robin, you always insisted we be equal partners in this endeavor and never made me feel anything less than that.

Thank you to everyone on Emily's team and at Penguin for helping me learn the book-writing process and patiently working through my deficiencies. Caroline and Ginny, you are such wonderful editors to work with—always helpful, positive, and encouraging. You two are like my editing parents! I also want to thank Ann Godoff, Scott Moyers, Matt Boyd, Danielle Plafsky, Elisabeth Calamari, Aly D'Amato, and Meg Gerrity.

I am fortunate to also have a wonderful day job, and I want to thank all the doctors, managers, and staff at Maternal Fetal Medicine Associates for putting up with me while I became an incorrigible author over the past year or so, and for dealing with my false sense of importance and celebrity.

To the other Emily in my life, Emily O'Connor, and the whole team at Digital Limelight Media in the great city of Grand Rapids, Michigan, thank you for overseeing my podcast and my work-related PR. You are a pleasure to work with, and hopefully this book will drive more traffic to our websites, so your annual numbers will look even better!

To my family and friends, thank you for encouraging me and letting me bore you with the details of this book, my podcast, my career, and Cubs baseball. Michal, thank you for your constant encouragement and for being the best wife, friend, and counsel anyone could ask for. Noam, Kira, Elan, Nili, and Mia, you are absolutely terrific children and no matter how busy I may seem, there is nothing in this world I enjoy more than spending time with you guys. I am blessed with loving and wonderful parents, Barbara and Jack Fox, and I am also lucky enough to have gained two more parents in my life, Marcelle and Saul Agus. I am so sad that Saul passed away eight years ago—he would have loved this book. A special thank you to Jack and Saul, also known as Dr. Jacob Fox and Dr. Saul G. Agus, as they were my inspiration to become a doctor those many years ago.

Finally, to my beloved patients. Thank you for allowing me to share in your happiest, and sometimes saddest, moments. I am deeply humbled and honored by your trust and I do not take it lightly. I cherish the bonds we have formed, and I am in awe of your strength. Thank you for letting me be a part of your lives. You are all a part of mine.

—Nathan Fox, MD

Appendix

Resources

More from Emily and Nate

Emily's Substack newsletter, *ParentData*: www.parentdata.org

Nate's podcast on pregnancy, birth, and women's health:
Healthful Woman: www.healthfulwoman.com

Resources on Racial Maternal and Infant Health Gaps

Chidi, Erica, and Erica P. Cahill. (2020). "Protecting Your Birth: A Guide for Black Mothers." *The New York Times*.

Cottom, T. M. (2019). *Thick: And Other Essays*. The New Press.

Geronimus, A. (2023). *Weathering: The Extraordinary Stress of Ordinary Life in an Unjust Society*. Little Brown Spark.

Opoku-Agyeman, A. (2022). *The Black Agenda: Bold Solutions for a Broken System*. St. Martin's Press.

Villarosa, L. (2022). *Under the Skin: The Hidden Toll of Racism on American Lives and on the Health of Our Nation*. Doubleday.

Notes

Part 2: Complications

1. Hoyert, D. L. "Maternal mortality rates in the United States, 2021." Centers for Disease Control and Prevention, 2023, https://www.cdc.gov/nchs/data/hestat/maternal-mortality/2021/maternal-mortality-rates-2021.pdf.

2. Kennedy-Moulton, K., et al. *Maternal and infant health inequality: New evidence from linked administrative data.* No. w30693. National Bureau of Economic Research, 2022.

3. Perry, J. C. "The Black maternal mortality rate in the US is an international crisis," *The Root*, September 30, 2016, https://www.theroot.com/the-black-maternal-mortality-rate-in-the-us-is-an-inter-1790857011.

4. Oster, E. "Black maternal health is maternal health: Dr. Quantrilla Ard on birthing while Black—and her search for answers," *ParentData*, April 11, 2023, https://parentdata.org/black-maternal-health-is-maternal-health.

Chapter 4: Hyperemesis Gravidarum

1. Dean, C. R., et al. "The chance of recurrence of hyperemesis gravidarum: A systematic review." *European Journal of Obstetrics and Gynecology and Reproductive Biology X* 5 (2020): 100105.

2. Trogstad, L. I., et al. "Recurrence risk in hyperemesis gravidarum." *BJOG* 112.12 (2005): 1641–1645.

3. Nurmi, M., et al. "Recurrence patterns of hyperemesis gravidarum." *American Journal of Obstetrics and Gynecology* 219.5 (2018): 469.e1–469.e10.

4. Fiaschi, L., et al. "Hospital admission for hyperemesis gravidarum: A nationwide study of occurrence, reoccurrence and risk factors among 8.2 million pregnancies." *Human Reproduction* 31.8 (2016): 1675–1684.

5. Fejzo, M. S., et al. "Recurrence risk of hyperemesis gravidarum." *Journal of Midwifery and Women's Health* 56.2 (2011): 132–136.

6. Trogstad et al. "Recurrence risk in hyperemesis gravidarum."

7. Nurmi et al. "Recurrence patterns of hyperemesis gravidarum."

8. Fejzo, M., et al. "GDF15 linked to maternal risk of nausea and vomiting during pregnancy." *Nature* 625.7996 (2024): 760–767.

9. Koren, G., and R. Cohen. "The use of cannabis for hyperemesis gravidarum (HG)." *Journal of Cannabis Research* 2.1 (2020): 1–4.

Chapter 5: First-Trimester Miscarriage

1. Ammon Avalos, L., et al. "A systematic review to calculate background miscarriage rates using life table analysis." *Birth Defects Research Part A: Clinical and Molecular Teratology* 94 (2012): 417–423.

2. Magnus, M. C., et al. "Role of maternal age and pregnancy history in risk of miscarriage: Prospective register based study." *BMJ* 364 (2019): l869.

3. Cohain, J. S., et al. "Spontaneous first trimester miscarriage rates per woman among parous women with 1 or more pregnancies of 24 weeks or more." *BMC Pregnancy Childbirth* 17 (2017): 437.

4. Naert, M. N., et al. "Stratified risk of pregnancy loss for women with a viable singleton pregnancy in the first trimester." *Journal of Maternal-Fetal and Neonatal Medicine* 35.23 (2022): 4491–4495.

5. American College of Obstetricians and Gynecologists. "Early pregnancy loss." *Clinical Practice Bulletin*, no. 200 (November 2018). https://www.acog.org/clinical/clinical-guidance/practice-bulletin/articles/2018/11/early-pregnancy-loss.

6. Acien, P. "Incidence of Müllerian defects in fertile and infertile women." *Human Reproduction* 12.7 (1997): 1372–1376.

7. Jacobs, P. A., et al. "Estimates of the frequency of chromosome abnormalities detectable in unselected newborns using moderate levels of banding." *Journal of Medical Genetics* 29.2 (1992): 103–108.

Chapter 6: Second-Trimester Miscarriage

1. Ammon Avalos, L., et al. "A systematic review to calculate background miscarriage rates using life table analysis." *Birth Defects Research Part A: Clinical and Molecular Teratology* 94 (2012): 417–423.

Chapter 7: Gestational Diabetes

1. Gregory, E. C. W., and D. M. Ely. "Trends and characteristics in gestational diabetes: United States, 2016–2020." *National Vital Statistics Reports* 71.3 (2022): 1–15.

2. American College of Obstetricians and Gynecologists. "ACOG practice bulletin no. 201: Pregestational diabetes mellitus." *Obstetrics and Gynecology* 132.6 (2018): e228–e248.

3. Kim, C., et al. "Recurrence of gestational diabetes mellitus: A systematic review." *Diabetes Care* 30.5 (2007): 1314–1319.

4. Schwartz, N., et al. "The prevalence of gestational diabetes mellitus recurrence—effect of ethnicity and parity: A metaanalysis." *American Journal of Obstetrics and Gynecology* 213.3 (2015): 310–317.

5. Chodick, G., et al. "The risk of overt diabetes mellitus among women with gestational diabetes: A population-based study." *Diabetic Medicine* 27.7 (2010): 779–785.

6. Guo, X. Y., et al. "Improving the effectiveness of lifestyle interventions for gestational diabetes prevention: A meta-analysis and meta-regression." *BJOG* 126.3 (2019): 311–320.

7. Makarem, N., et al. "Association of a Mediterranean diet pattern with adverse pregnancy outcomes among US women." *JAMA Network Open* 5.12 (2022): e2248165.

8. Vanky, E., et al. "Metformin versus placebo from first trimester to delivery in polycystic ovary syndrome: A randomized, controlled multicenter study." *Journal of Clinical Endocrinology and Metabolism* 95.12 (2010): E448–455.

9. Li, L., et al. "Myo-inositol supplementation for the prevention of gestational diabetes: A meta-analysis of randomized controlled trials." *European Journal of Obstetrics and Gynecology and Reproductive Biology* 273 (2022): 38–43.

Chapter 8: Preeclampsia

1. Bartsch, E., et al. "Clinical risk factors for pre-eclampsia determined in early pregnancy: Systematic review and meta-analysis of large cohort studies." *BMJ* 353 (2016): i1753.

2. The Fetal Medicine Foundation. "Risk for preeclampsia." https://fetalmedi cine.org/research/assess/preeclampsia/first-trimester (accessed June 20, 2023).

3. Duley, L., et al. "Antiplatelet agents for preventing pre-eclampsia and its complications." *Cochrane Database of Systematic Reviews* 10 (2019): CD004659.

4. Woo Kinshella, M. L., et al. "Calcium for pre-eclampsia prevention: A systematic review and network meta-analysis to guide personalised antenatal care." *BJOG* 129.11 (2022): 1833–1843.

Chapter 9: Fetal Growth Restriction

1. Voskamp, B. J., et al. "Recurrence of small-for-gestational-age pregnancy: Analysis of first and subsequent singleton pregnancies in the Netherlands." *American Journal of Obstetrics and Gynecology* 208.5 (2013): 374.e1–6.

2. Ananth, C. V., et al. "Recurrence of fetal growth restriction in singleton and twin gestations." *Journal of Maternal-Fetal and Neonatal Medicine* 22.8 (2009): 654–661.

3. Surkan, P. J., et al. "Previous preterm and small-for-gestational-age births and the subsequent risk of stillbirth." *New England Journal of Medicine* 350.8 (2004): 777–785.

4. Auger, N., et al. "The joint influence of marital status, interpregnancy interval, and neighborhood on small for gestational age birth: A retrospective cohort study." *BMC Pregnancy and Childbirth* 8 (2008): 1–9; Shults, Ruth A., et al. "Effects of short interpregnancy intervals on small-for-gestational age and preterm births." *Epidemiology* 10.3 (1999): 250–254.

5. Thorsdottir, I., and B. E. Birgisdottir. "Different weight gain in women of normal weight before pregnancy: Postpartum weight and birth weight." *Obstetrics and Gynecology* 92.3 (1998): 377–383.

6. Crovetto, F., et al. "Effects of Mediterranean diet or mindfulness-based stress reduction on prevention of small-for-gestational age birth weights in newborns born to at-risk pregnant individuals: The IMPACT BCN randomized clinical trial." *JAMA* 326.21 (2021): 2150–2160.

Chapter 10: Preterm Birth

1. "Natality Information: Live Births." Centers for Disease Control and Prevention. https://wonder.cdc.gov/natality.html (last updated October 3, 2023).

2. Lykke, J. A., et al. "Recurring complications in second pregnancy." *Obstetrics and Gynecology* 113.6 (2009): 1217–1224.

3. Yamashita, M., et al. "Incidence and risk factors for recurrent spontaneous preterm birth: A retrospective cohort study in Japan." *Journal of Obstetrics and Gynaecology Research* 41.11 (2015): 1708–1714.

4. Laughon, S. K., et al. "The NICHD Consecutive Pregnancies Study: Recurrent preterm delivery by subtype." *American Journal of Obstetrics and Gynecology* 210.2 (2014): 131.e1–8.

5. Mercer, B. M., et al. "The preterm prediction study: Effect of gestational age and cause of preterm birth on subsequent obstetric outcome." *American Journal of Obstetrics and Gynecology* 181.5 (1999): 1216–1221.

6. Marinovich, M. L., et al. "Associations between interpregnancy interval and preterm birth by previous preterm birth status in four high-income countries: A cohort study." *BJOG* 128.7 (2021): 1134–1143.

7. Hanley, G. E., et al. "Interpregnancy interval and adverse pregnancy outcomes: An analysis of successive pregnancies." *Obstetrics and Gynecology* 129.3 (2017): 408–415; Ball, S. J., et al. "Re-evaluation of link between interpregnancy interval and adverse birth outcomes: Retrospective cohort study matching two intervals per mother." *BMJ* 349 (2014): g4333.

8. Menzies, R., et al. "Risk of singleton preterm birth after prior twin preterm birth: A systematic review and meta-analysis." *American Journal of Obstetrics and Gynecology* 223.2 (2020): 204.e1–204.e8.

9. McGoldrick, E., et al. "Antenatal corticosteroids for accelerating fetal lung maturation for women at risk of preterm birth." *Cochrane Database of Systematic Reviews* 12.12 (2020): CD004454.

10. Meis, P. J., et al. "Prevention of recurrent preterm delivery by 17 alpha-hydroxyprogesterone caproate." *New England Journal of Medicine* 348.24 (2003): 2379–2385.

11. Blackwell, S. C., et al. "17-OHPC to prevent recurrent preterm birth in singleton gestations (PROLONG study): A multicenter, international, randomized double-blind trial." *American Journal of Perinatology* 37.2 (2020): 127–136.

12. EPPPIC Group. "Evaluating Progestogens for Preventing Preterm birth International Collaborative (EPPPIC): Meta-analysis of individual participant data from randomised controlled trials." *Lancet* 397.10280 (2021): 1183–1194.

13. Murphy, C. C., et al. "In utero exposure to 17α-hydroxyprogesterone caproate and risk of cancer in offspring." *American Journal of Obstetrics and Gynecology* 226.1 (2022): 132.e1–132.e14.

14. Alfirevic, Z., et al. "Cervical stitch (cerclage) for preventing preterm birth in singleton pregnancy." *Cochrane Database of Systematic Reviews* 6.6 (2017): CD008991.

15. Landman, A. J. E. M. C., et al. "Evaluation of low-dose aspirin in the prevention of recurrent spontaneous preterm labour (the APRIL study): A multicentre, randomised, double-blinded, placebo-controlled trial." *PLOS Medicine* 19.2 (2022): e1003892.

16. Middleton, P., et al. "Omega-3 fatty acid addition during pregnancy." *Cochrane Database of Systematic Reviews* 11.11 (2018): CD003402.

17. Sosa, C. G., et al. "Bed rest in singleton pregnancies for preventing preterm birth." *Cochrane Database of Systematic Reviews* 2015.3 (2015): CD003581.

18. Grobman, W. A., et al. "Activity restriction among women with a short cervix." *Obstetrics and Gynecology* 121.6 (2013): 1181–1186.

19. Urquhart, C., et al. "Home uterine monitoring for detecting preterm labour." *Cochrane Database of Systematic Reviews* 2.2 (2017): CD006172.

Chapter 11: Cesarean Section (and VBAC)

1. Whyte, H., et al. "Outcomes of children at 2 years after planned cesarean birth versus planned vaginal birth for breech presentation at term: The International Randomised Term Breech Trial." *American Journal of Obstetrics and Gynecology* 191.3 (2004): 864–871.

2. Oonagh, E. K., et al. "Long-term risks and benefits associated with cesarean delivery for mother, baby, and subsequent pregnancies: Systematic review and meta-analysis." *PLOS Medicine* 15.1 (2018): e1002494.

3. McMahon, M. J., et al. "Comparison of a trial of labor with an elective second cesarean section." *New England Journal of Medicine* 335 (1996): 689–695.

4. Thirukumar, P., et al. "Women's experiences of intrapartum care and recovery in relation to planned caesarean sections: An interview study." *Women and Birth* 34.3 (2021): e248–e254.

5. Shorten, A., et al. "The importance of mode of birth after previous cesarean: Success, satisfaction, and postnatal health." *Journal of Midwifery and Women's Health* 57.2 (2012): 126–132.

6. Blomquist, J. L., et al. "Mothers' satisfaction with planned vaginal and planned cesarean birth." *American Journal of Perinatology* 28.5 (2011): 383–388.

7. Dodd, J. M., et al. "Planned elective repeat caesarean section versus planned vaginal birth for women with a previous caesarean birth." *Cochrane Database of Systematic Reviews* 12 (2013): CD004224.

8. Martin, J. A., et al. "Births in the United States, 2021." Centers for Disease Control and Prevention, NCHS data brief no. 442 (August 2022). https://www.cdc.gov/nchs/products/databriefs/db442.htm#section_3.

9. Grobman, W. A., et al. "Prediction of vaginal birth after cesarean delivery in term gestations: A calculator without race and ethnicity." *American Journal of Obstetrics and Gynecology* 225.6 (2021): 664.E1–664.E7.

10. Maternal-Fetal Medicine Units Network. "Vaginal birth after cesarean." https://mfmunetwork.bsc.gwu.edu/web/mfmunetwork/vaginal-birth-after-cesarean-calculator (accessed June 20, 2023).

11. Baradaran, K. "Risk of uterine rupture with vaginal birth after cesarean in twin gestations." *Obstetrics and Gynecology International* (2021): 6693142.

12. Fitzpatrick, K. E., et al. "Uterine rupture by intended mode of delivery in the UK: A national case-control study." *PLOS Medicine* 9.3 (2012): e1001184.

13. Silver, R. M., et al. "Maternal morbidity associated with multiple repeat cesarean deliveries." *Obstetrics and Gynecology* 107.6 (2006): 1226–1232.

14. Keag, O. E., et al. "Long-term risks and benefits associated with cesarean delivery for mother, baby, and subsequent pregnancies: Systematic review and meta-analysis." *PLOS Medicine* 15.1 (2018): e1002494.

Chapter 12: Severe Maternal Morbidity

1. Sheldon, W. R., et al. "Postpartum haemorrhage management, risks, and maternal outcomes: Findings from the World Health Organization Multicountry Survey on Maternal and Newborn Health." *BJOG* 121 (2014): Suppl 1:5–13.

2. Oberg, A. S., et al. "Patterns of recurrence of postpartum hemorrhage in a large population-based cohort." *American Journal of Obstetrics and Gynecology* 210.3 (2014): 229.e1–8.

3. Lamy, C., et al. "Ischemic stroke in young women: Risk of recurrence during subsequent pregnancies. French Study Group on Stroke in Pregnancy." *Neurology* 55.2 (2000): 269–274.

4. McColl, M. D., et al. "Risk factors for pregnancy associated venous thromboembolism." *Journal of Thrombosis and Haemostasis* 78.4 (1997): 1183–1188.

5. de Moreuil, C., et al. "Risk factors for recurrence during a pregnancy following a first venous thromboembolism: A French observational study." *Journal of Thrombosis and Haemostasis* 20.4 (2022): 909–918.

6. Bauer, M. E., et al. "Maternal sepsis mortality and morbidity during hospitalization for delivery: Temporal trends and independent associations for severe sepsis." *Anesthesia and Analgesia* 117.4 (2013): 944–950.

Chapter 13: Stillbirth

1. American College of Obstetricians and Gynecologists et al. "Management of Stillbirth: Obstetric Care Consensus No. 10." *Obstetrics and Gynecology* 135.3 (2020): e110–e132.

2. Lamont, K., et al. "Risk of recurrent stillbirth: Systematic review and meta-analysis." *BMJ* 350 (2015): 3080.

3. Wennerholm, U., et al. "Induction of labour at 41 weeks versus expectant management and induction of labour at 42 weeks (SWEdish Post-term Induction Study, SWEPIS): Multicentre, open label, randomised, superiority trial." *BMJ* 367 (2019): l6131.

4. Grobman, W. A., et al. "Labor induction versus expectant management in low-risk nulliparous women." *New England Journal of Medicine* 379.6 (2018): 513–523.

5. Bellussi, F., et al. "Fetal movement counting and perinatal mortality: A systematic review and meta-analysis." *Obstetrics and Gynecology* 135.2 (2020): 453–462.

6. Norman, J. E., et al. "Awareness of fetal movements and care package to reduce fetal mortality (AFFIRM): A stepped wedge, cluster-randomised trial." *Lancet* 392.10158 (2018): 1629–1638.

7. Derwig, I. E., et al. "Association of placental volume measured by MRI and birth weight percentile." *Journal of Magnetic Resonance Imaging* 34.5 (2011): 1125–1130.

8. Azpurua, H., et al. "Determination of placental weight using two-dimensional sonography and volumetric mathematic modeling." *American Journal of Perinatology* 27 (2009): 151–155.

Chapter 14: Recovery Complications

1. Smith, L. A., et al. "Incidence of and risk factors for perineal trauma: A prospective observational study." *BMC Pregnancy Childbirth* 13.59 (2013).

2. Jiang, H., et al. "Selective versus routine use of episiotomy for vaginal birth." *Cochrane Database of Systematic Reviews* (2017): CD000081.

3. Yogev, Y., et al. "Third and fourth degree perineal tears—the risk of recurrence in subsequent pregnancy." *Journal of Maternal-Fetal and Neonatal Medicine* 27.2 (2014): 177–181.

4. Payne, T. N., et al. "Prior third- or fourth-degree perineal tears and recurrence risks." *International Journal of Gynecology and Obstetrics* 64.1 (1999): 55–57.

5. Priddis, H., et al. "Risk of recurrence, subsequent mode of birth and morbidity for women who experienced severe perineal trauma in a first birth in New South Wales between 2000–2008: A population based data linkage study." *BMC Pregnancy Childbirth* 13 (2013): 89.

6. Aquino, C. I., et al. "Perineal massage during labor: A systematic review and meta-analysis of randomized controlled trials." *Journal of Maternal-Fetal and Neonatal Medicine* 33.6 (2020): 1051–1063.

7. Aasheim, V., et al. "Perineal techniques during the second stage of labour for reducing perineal trauma." *Cochrane Database of Systematic Reviews* 6.6 (2017): CD006672.

8. Barber, M. D., and C. Maher. "Epidemiology and outcome assessment of pelvic organ prolapse." *International Urogynecology Journal* 24.11 (2013): 1783–1790.

9. Nygaard, I., et al. "Prevalence of symptomatic pelvic floor disorders in US women." *JAMA* 300.11 (2008): 1311–1316.

10. Kawakita, T., et al. "Surgical site infections after cesarean delivery: Epidemiology, prevention and treatment." *Maternal Health, Neonatology and Perinatology* 3.12 (2017).

Chapter 15: Postpartum Mental Health Conditions

1. Viguera, A. "Postpartum unipolar major depression: Epidemiology, clinical features, assessment, and diagnosis." UpToDate, https://www.uptodate.com

/contents/postpartum-unipolar-major-depression-epidemiology-clinical-features-assessment-and-diagnosis (accessed January 24, 2023).

2. Viguera, "Postpartum unipolar major depression."

3. Rasmussen, M. H., et al. "Risk, treatment duration, and recurrence risk of postpartum affective disorder in women with no prior psychiatric history: A population-based cohort study." *PLOS Medicine* 14.9 (2017): e1002392.

4. O'Connor, E., et al. "Primary care screening for and treatment of depression in pregnant and postpartum women: Evidence report and systematic review for the US Preventive Services Task Force." *JAMA* 315.4 (2016): 388–406.

Chapter 16: Breastfeeding Barriers

1. Brownell, E., et al. "Delayed onset lactogenesis II predicts the cessation of any or exclusive breastfeeding." *Journal of Pediatrics* 161.4 (2012): 608–614.

2. Institute of Medicine (US) Committee on Nutritional Status During Pregnancy and Lactation. *Nutrition During Lactation.* Washington, DC: National Academies Press, 1991, https://doi.org/10.17226/1577.

3. Institute of Medicine (US) Committee on Nutritional Status During Pregnancy and Lactation, *Nutrition During Lactation.*

4. Puapornpong, P., et al. "Nipple pain incidence, the predisposing factors, the recovery period after care management, and the exclusive breastfeeding outcome." *Breastfeeding Medicine* 12.3 (2017): 169–173.

5. Ureño, T. L., et al. "Dysphoric milk ejection reflex: A descriptive study." *Breastfeeding Medicine* 14.9 (2019): 666–673.

Index

NOTE: *Italic page numbers indicate charts*

chromosomal translocation, 63–64, 66
clindamycin, 132
Cochrane Review, 102, 129–30, 132,
    144–45
cognitive therapy, 51
colectomies, 120
compounding pharmacies, 127, 128
counting kicks, 180, 183, 184, 188
COVID vaccines, 27
Crear-Perry, Joia, 37
Cribsheet (Oster), 214
C-sections. *See* cesarean sections
cytomegalovirus (CMV), 175

Danish study, 124–25, 208–9
data, xvii–xviii
    fact finding, 9–10, 15–17
    recurrence risks and, 31–36. *See also*
        recurrence risks
deep vein thrombosis (DVT), 165–66
dehydration and hyperemesis
    gravidarum, 43, 44, 50, 51–52
delayed lactogenesis, 213, 215–16
"delivery summary," 17
depression. *See also* postpartum
    depression
    bed rest and, 132
diabetes
    gestational. *See* gestational diabetes
    indicated preterm births and, 134
    before pregnancy, 85, 86–87, 89
diet
    for gestational diabetes, 90–91, *91*, 93
    for small for gestational age, 113,
        114–15
dilation and aspiration (D&A), 74
dilation and curettage (D&C), 74–75
dilation and evacuation (D&E), 74–75
*Dobbs v. Jackson Women's Health
    Organization*, 38
Down syndrome, 174
doxylamine, 51
dysphoric milk ejection reflex (D-MER),
    218

E. coli, 175
early stillbirths, 173–74. *See also*
    stillbirths

eclampsia, 98
Edinburgh Postnatal Depression Scale,
    204–5
ejection reflex issues, 218–20
emotional preparations, 5–10
    step 1: frame the question, 7–8
    step 2: fact find, 9–10
    step 3: final decision, 10
    step 4: follow-up, 10
energy loss and hyperemesis
    gravidarum, 43, 44
epidurals, xx
episiotomies, 194, 199–200, 201
exercise
    for gestational diabetes, 90–91
    for preeclampsia, 99, 103
Expecting Better (Oster), xiv, xv, xx

fact finding, 9–10, 15–17
Factor V Leiden, 176
Family Firm, The (Oster), 7
fault, questions of, 23–24
FDA (Food and Drug Administration)
    Center for Drug Evaluation and
        Research, 128
    Makena progesterone, 127–28
    preeclampsia blood test, 103–4
    Zuranalone, 209
fetal echocardiograms and
    preeclampsia, 94
fetal growth assessments, 106–7
fetal growth restriction (FGR), 109–17,
    176, 179
    bottom line, 117
    definition, 109, 110, 113
    medical perspective, 113–16
    recurrence risks, 109, 111, *116*
    SGA vs., 110–11
    uterine septum, 63
fetal hypothalamic-pituitary-adrenal
    axis, 135
Finnish register study, 47–48
first-degree vaginal tears, 193
first-trimester complications, 43–68
    hyperemesis gravidarum. *See*
        hyperemesis gravidarum
    miscarriages. *See* first-trimester
        miscarriages

saline infusion sonohysterograms (SIS), 66–67, 81–82, 183
script preparations, 21–28
 question 1: what happened?, 22–23
 question 2: why did it happen to me?, 23–24
 question 3: is it going to happen to me again?, 25–27
 question 4: what can be done to prevent it from happening again?, 27–28
second-degree vaginal tears, 193
second-trimester miscarriages, 71–83
 bottom line, 83
 cases, 72–73, 75–77
 definition, 71, 73–74
 medical perspective, 78–82
 overall prevalence, 71–73, 72
 recurrence risks, 71, 77–78
selfishness, 187
sepsis, 167–68
 recurrence and prevention, 168
17-OHPC (17-OH progesterone), 126, 128–29, 137
severe maternal morbidity, 4, 159–72
 blood clots, 165–66
 bottom line, 172
 cases, 160–61
 definition, 159
 medical perspective, 168–72
 overall prevalence, 159–60
 peripartum cardiomyopathy, 166–67
 postpartum hemorrhage, 162–63
 sepsis, 167–68
 strokes, 163–64
severe preeclampsia, 98–99, 101, 108
sex
 abstaining after miscarriages, 62
 painful, recovery complications, 193
SGA. See small for gestational age
shampoo ads, 32, 33, 34
shoulder dystocia, 87
sleep and postpartum depression, 204, 205, 209
small for gestational age (SGA), 109–17
 bottom line, 117
 definition, 109, 110, 113
 FGR vs., 110–11

medical perspective, 113–16
prevention, 112–13
recurrence risks, 109, 111, 116
smoking, 24, 48, 110, 112, 114
spontaneous preterm births, 119–20, 134–36
steroids, 103, 125
stillbirths, 173–88
 bottom line, 188
 definition, 173–74
 medical perspective, 181–88
 overall prevalence, 173–74
 prevention, 178–81
 recurrence risks, 173, 175–78, 188
stress, 113, 116, 180, 185, 216
strokes, 163–64
 recurrence and treatment, 164
Summers, Kaleigh, 221–22
support network, 186–87
 emotional preparations, 8, 9
sutures, 169, 197
Swedish studies, 162, 179
switching providers, 12–13
systemic racism, 37–38

Tay-Sachs disease, 19
testing. See also blood tests; genetic testing
 autosomal genetic conditions, 18–20
 first-trimester miscarriages, 66–67
 genetic carrier screenings, 17–19, 82, 183
 gestational diabetes, 85–88
 possible additional, 17–19
 preimplantation genetic testing, 19, 64
Thick (Cottom), 38
third-degree vaginal tears, 193
thrombophilia, 82, 176–77, 183, 184
timing the delivery, 7–8, 184–85
total parenteral nutrition (TPN), 52
traumatic birth. See severe maternal morbidity
treatments, xviii, 32, 33–34. See also specific treatments
 for antiphospholipid antibody syndrome, 67, 82
 costs and insurance considerations, 14–15

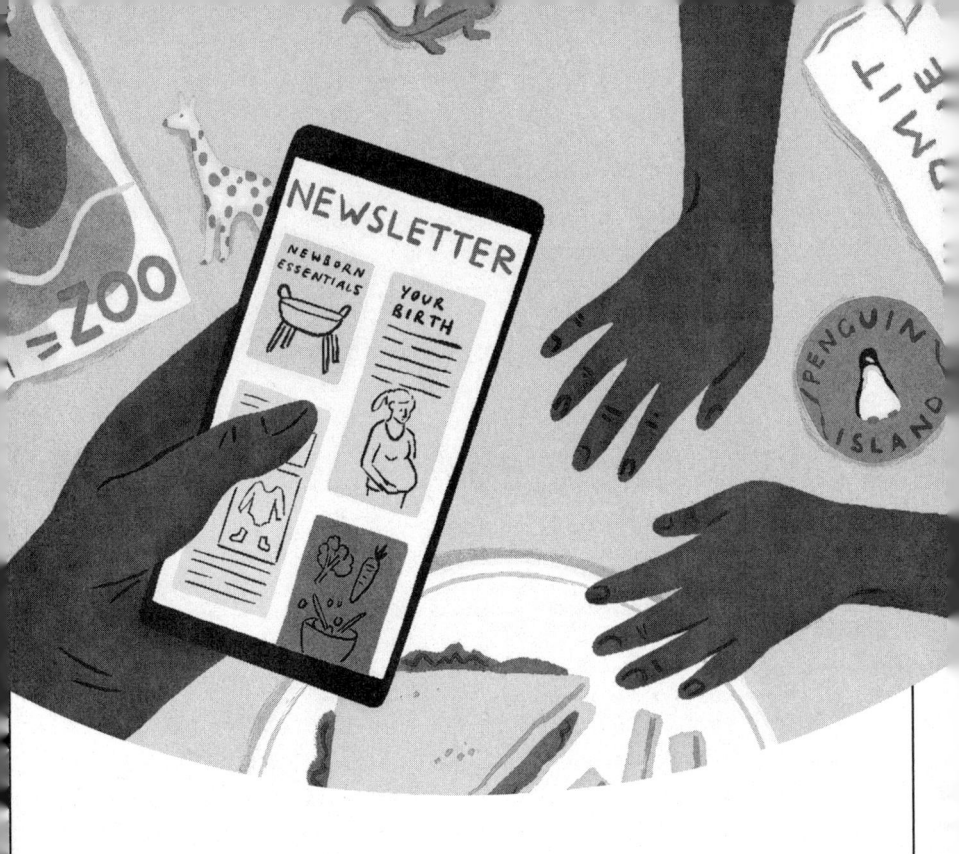

Have more questions about navigating pregnancy and parenting?

Need the reassurance and data that you didn't get from
your one a.m. panic Google?

Want to ask Emily Oster your questions and connect
with other readers?

ParentData is a data-driven guide through pregnancy, parenthood,
and beyond created by Emily Oster. Visit parentdata.org for
up-to-the-minute research and thousands of articles with answers
to the questions you have in your daily life.